Laboratory Procedures for
Inlays, Crowns and Bridges

General Series Editor

J. M. Mumford

Laboratory Procedures for
Inlays, Crowns and Bridges

DEREK STANANOUGHT *FBIST*

Certificate in Dental Technology
Certificate in Dental Ceramics, Crown and Bridge Work
of the City and Guild of London Institute

Lecturer in Dental Technology
John Dalton Faculty of Technology
Manchester Polytechnic

(*formerly* Instructor in Crown and Bridge Techniques
School of Dental Surgery, University of Liverpool)

Edited by

J. M. MUMFORD
PhD MSc LDS(Liv) MS(Mich) FDSRCS(Eng)

Reader in Operative Dental Surgery
University of Liverpool

Consultant Dental Surgeon
Liverpool Area Health Authority (Teaching)

Blackwell Scientific Publications
Oxford London Edinburgh Melbourne

ISBN 0 632 00791 5

First published 1975

Distributed in the U.S.A. by
J. B. Lippincott Company, Philadelphia

and in Canada by
J. B. Lippincott Company of Canada Ltd, Toronto

Set in 11 Photon Times

Printed in Great Britain
at the Alden Press, Oxford

Contents

Editor's foreword

This book is unpretentious, the author presenting his material in a clear straightforward manner which will help the reader to carry out the procedures described. It is clearly a workshop manual and should always be kept at hand, especially by students of the subject, whether they be dental students or student technicians. In addition it will be helpful to dentists and qualified technicians wishing to be reminded of detail or brought up to date with these techniques.

It is no part of a technician's job to encroach on the clinician's territory and the author is careful to avoid trespassing in this way. The few statements made on clinical matters have been designed solely to provide a link between the chairside and the laboratory.

I am sure the book will be found very helpful by all who read it.

J. M. MUMFORD

Preface

The aim of this book is to instruct undergraduate dental students and dental technicians in the technical procedures involved when making inlays, crowns and bridges. It is assumed that the reader has a little knowledge of dental laboratory procedures coupled with a general understanding of the anatomy of the mouth, including tooth morphology.

The text has not been written with references, but some are given in the appendix where it is felt that special mention is warranted. Some recommended readings are also given for those wishing to study the theoretical aspects of the techniques described.

As with any craft there are many ways of attaining the same end. The techniques described are by no means the only methods available, but they have been proved successful repeatedly over many years.

I wish to thank Dr J.M. Mumford for the encouragement and advice he has given throughout the preparation of this book. My thanks also to Mr R.W. Williams and Mr B.A. Tabberer, Dental Instructors of Birmingham University, for reading the manuscript and giving their advice.

DEREK STANANOUGHT

1 Construction of Casts

All technical procedures commence with an impression of the patient's dentition. The most commonly-used impression materials are compound, rubber base and irreversible hydrocolloids (alginate), but use is also made of reversible hydrocolloids, zinc oxide—eugenol and plaster of Paris. An impression of a single preparation is often taken in impression compound supported by a copper ring, an alginate impression of the whole dentition being taken at the same sitting for localizing purposes. Rubber base, whilst extremely accurate, is also costly, so it is generally reserved for taking impressions of multiple preparations. Upper and lower alginate impressions are taken to produce study casts, which assist the dental surgeon in diagnosis and treatment planning.

STUDY CASTS

Study casts may be used to:

a Facilitate full analysis of the occlusion (when articulated)
b Help the dental surgeon to analyse the feasibility of various restorations
c Provide a basis for waxing restorative measures such as full mouth rehabilitation and complex bridge designs
d Record permanently the patient's dentition
e Help the dentist to discuss possible treatments with the technician and patient
f Construct special, closely-adapted trays upon them.

Pouring and trimming of study casts is carried out in the following manner.

1 The casts are poured, care being taken to vibrate the dental stone slowly along the floor of the impression to minimize air inclusions.

1

When the cast has set, a base is made using an equal mixture of dental stone and plaster of Paris, a disposable mould of plastic being useful for forming this. The base is allowed to set for 1 hour before attempting to remove the cast from the impression.

2   The occlusal surface of the lower cast is placed upon a block of wood, approximately 8 cm high by 30 cm square, with the heels and the last molar overhanging the edge of the block, to allow for the Curve of Spee. Onto the wood is also placed an engineer's scribing block, the pointer of which is set at 1½× the anatomical height of the lower cast (Fig. 1.1). A line is scribed around the base of the cast and the cast trimmed to the line on an electric trimmer.

3   The upper and lower casts are occluded and the base of the lower cast placed on the block. The height of the pointer of the scribing block is adjusted to double the previous height, the base of the upper cast is marked and trimmed to the mark (Fig. 1.2).

4   Two pencil marks, about 5 cm apart, are made down the centre of the palate of the upper cast and the 90°-angle line of a plastic protractor placed along the two marks with the lower border of the protractor 5 mm behind the two tuberosities and the cast marked (Fig. 1.3). When the posterior border has been trimmed the casts are re-occluded and the position of the posterior border of the upper marked on the lower cast, which is then trimmed to this mark.

Fig. 1.1 The occlusal surface of the lower cast is placed on a block of wood with the heels and last molar overhanging the edge of the block. The base of the cast is marked using an engineer's scribing block (A). (B) Anatomical height of the cast.

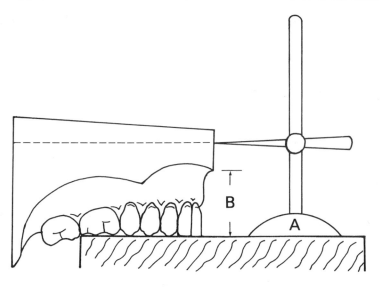

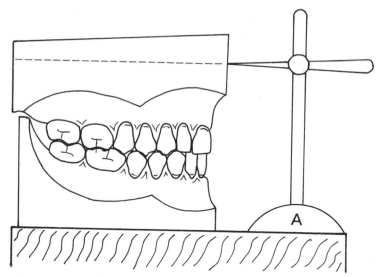

Fig. 1.2 After occlusion of the casts the height of the pointer is adjusted to double the previous height (Fig. 1.1) and the base of the upper cast scribed.

The casts are again occluded, placed on the electric trimmer and both posterior borders carefully trimmed level. It is then possible to occlude the casts accurately by placing them together on their posterior bases (Fig. 1.4).

5 The sides of the casts are trimmed independently to follow the line of the posterior teeth. The anterior region of the lower cast is curved from canine to canine, whilst both sides of the upper cast are angled from canine to the midline (Fig. 1.5).

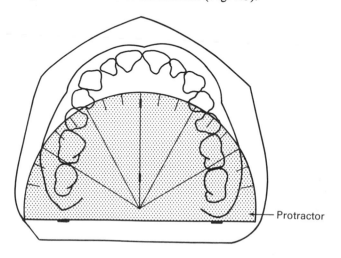

Fig. 1.3 A plastic protractor is used to mark the posterior border of the upper cast.

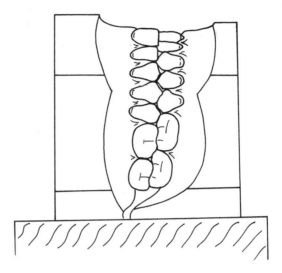

Fig. 1.4 After trimming it is possible to occlude the casts accurately by placing them together on their posterior bases.

WORKING CASTS

Before the construction of working casts is described it should be understood that the cast of a prepared tooth is called the die and it is accurately positioned in the master cast of the surrounding dentition. This die must be an accurate duplicate of the prepared tooth, be dimensionally stable and have a high surface hardness. The most popular materials are electrolytically deposited copper and die stones. Copper deposition is generally confined to compound impressions, whereas die stones are used in conjunction with rubber-base impressions.

Electrodeposition of compound impressions

A compound impression is taken in a carefully contoured copper ring. Most operators find it easy to use and reasonably accurate and stable. Only one die can be made from the material since it is destroyed when removed from the die. A separate full mouth alginate impression is also taken to localize the die in a cast of the surrounding dentition. Although wax or zinc oxide–eugenol occlusal registrations can be used, the full mouth localizing impression is

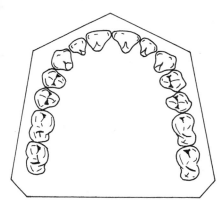

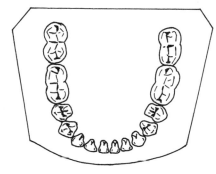

Fig. 1.5 The sides of the casts are trimmed to follow the line of the posterior teeth. The anterior region of the lower cast is curved whilst both sides of the upper cast are angled from canine to midline.

preferred, because it produces a definite localization, accurately records the dentition and makes mounting of casts on an articulator easier and more accurate. Alginate is sufficiently accurate for this purpose if the impression is covered with a damp cloth and placed in a selfseal polythene bag to prevent loss of moisture whilst the die is being constructed. The impression will remain sufficiently accurate for 24 hours.

Copper deposition is accomplished by placing the compound-copper ring impression in a bath containing a copper sulphate solution (see Appendix) and passing a small electric current through the solution and impression. In 12 hours the impression is coated with about 0.5 mm of pure copper. Excess impression compound on the outer surface of the copper ring is generally removed by the dental surgeon at the chairside so that if the impression is damaged during its removal a new impression may be taken without delay.

1 Blood and other debris is washed out of the impression which is dried under compressed air (see Appendix). The outer surface of the copper ring and both ends of a short piece of wire (the electrode) are cleaned, using sandpaper or a file. One end of the electrode is attached to the outer surface of the copper ring by wrapping it around the ring and twisting it tight or by using wax.

2 As impression compound is not a conductor of electricity it is coated with an electroconductive medium such as colloidal graphite (Aquadag) which must also contact the copper ring (see Appendix). This is dried with compressed air.

3 Deposition of copper on the copper ring and electrode is prevented by wrapping a piece of carding wax around them both and extending it 2 mm beyond the periphery of the impression to prevent excessive build up of copper in this area (Fig. 1.6).

4 Using a pipette, electrolyte (of copper sulphate solution) is dripped into the impression, care being taken not to trap air bubbles which prevent electrodeposition. If air is trapped the electrolyte is shaken out and the impression refilled until the base of the impression can be seen clearly through the electrolyte.

5 The free end of the electrode is attached to the electrical terminal (cathode) on the side of the bath and the current switched on. Failure to obtain a reading on the milliammeter usually means that one of

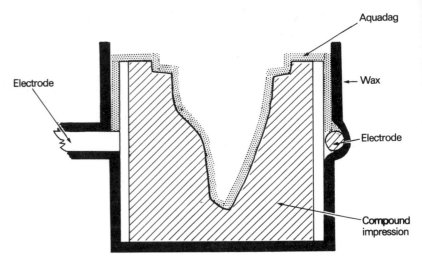

Fig. 1.6 Compound impression prepared for electrodeposition.

the above steps has been carried out incorrectly, in which case the impression is dried and the sequences repeated, checking all contacts.

6 The current is adjusted to 10–15 milliamps; a lower current produces a hard layer of copper but is slower to deposit; a higher current deposits quickly but the copper deposition is soft. A current of 10–15 mA maintained for at least 12 hours deposits approximately 0·5 mm thickness of copper, which is satisfactory. Deposition commences at the periphery of the impression, progressing slowly to the top of the cusps; the whole of the impression should be covered with copper by the end of an hour. If large areas remain free of deposition, the impression is washed and dried and the above sequences repeated.

7 Upon completion of the deposition period, the impression is removed from the electrolyte, thoroughly washed under cold running water and the protective wax and electrode removed from the copper ring, which is then dried.

8 To complete the die, the copper is backed with a hard material, such as autopolymerizing acrylic resin, to prevent it being damaged and to form a stump for holding and localizing purposes. A plastic dowel pin is trimmed so that the thinner end is about 2 mm longer than the depth of the impression. Autopolymerizing acrylic resin is mixed in a Dappen's glass and, whilst it is in the liquid state, a Le Cron carver is used either to vibrate or push small increments

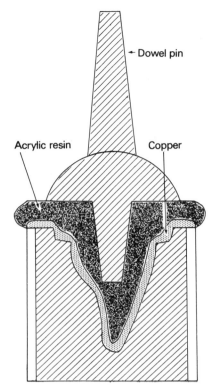

Fig. 1.7 The copper is backed with autopolymerizing acrylic resin and a plastic dowel pin inserted into it.

into the deposited copper. It is essential that air is not trapped between the resin and the copper because unsupported copper will collapse in use. As the resin polymerizes it is built to a height of 2 mm above the periphery of the impression. Acrylic resin is also added around the trimmed post of the dowel pin which is then inserted into the resin in the impression (Fig. 1.7). If this is carried out when the resin is turning to a 'dough', the pin will stand vertically in it until the resin has polymerized.

9 When polymerization is complete, the copper ring is gently warmed over a Bunsen burner flame to soften the compound which is then removed from the die. Overheating of compound should be avoided as this will make it stick to the die. Aquadag is removed from the surface of the die by washing with liquid soap.

10 Excess metal and acrylic resin are removed, using a pink alumina stone, to expose the true margin of the preparation and to facilitate the removal of the die from the master cast. When the copper becomes hot through friction, the die is quenched in water to prevent if coming away from the resin backing. The copper around the cusps is smoothed and the resin and bulbous portion of the dowel pin trimmed to form a taper from the margins of the preparation to the apex of the die (Fig. 1.8). It is important not to damage the smooth surface of the dowel pin whilst trimming because this causes unevenness which can prevent the removal of the die from the master cast.

11 A different method of trimming the die is used when a porcelain jacket crown is to be formed. The excess metal around the margins is removed until there is no sign of a false margin. The first 4 mm of the stump beyond the margin is trimmed with an outward taper of a few degrees and then tapered apically (Fig. 1.9). This allows the formation of an apron on the platinum matrix (Chapter 5).

Localizing the die

1 The localizing alginate impression is removed from the polythene bag, dried and the die positioned in the impression. After checking for fit it is removed.

2 A strip of carding wax is wrapped around and sealed to the tray to box the impression. The die is lightly lubricated with petroleum

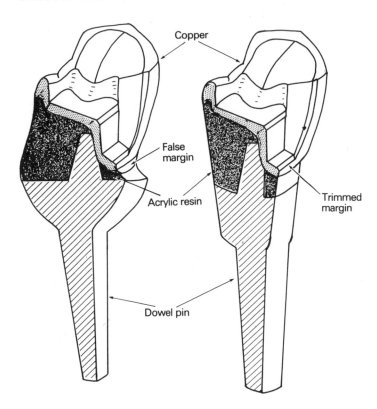

Fig. 1.8 The copper and resin are trimmed to remove the false margin and to form a tapered die.

jelly (Vaseline), slight excess being left around the periphery of the margins so when the die is firmly seated into the impression the jelly seals the periphery of the die and prevents plaster being vibrated into this part of the preparation. When the die has been firmly positioned into the impression a piece of 1 mm diameter wire is pressed into the carding wax to span the impression. The wire must be positioned so that light is visible between it and the dowel pin but it must not touch or dislodge the pin which is waxed to the wire.

3   An equal mix of plaster of Paris and Kaffir 'D' is vibrated into the impression and allowed to set for 1 hour, after which the carding wax, wire and impression are removed and the master cast trimmed on an electric trimmer.

4   A little plaster is removed from around the apex of the die and, by the use of the curved end of a large wax knife on the apex, the die is gently pushed out of the cast in an occlusal direction.

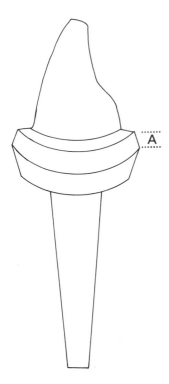

Fig. 1.9 Die for a porcelain jacket crown. The first 4 mm of the die (A) past the shoulder are given an outward taper.

5 To remove the die of a porcelain jacket crown from a master cast the plaster around the neck of the die must be removed, since the die is outwardly tapered in this region. This is done by making short saw cuts, with a piercing saw blade (fret saw), down the proximal areas to a depth of 6 mm and, using a flat sculptor, the labial and lingual gingival plaster is removed (Fig. 1.10). The proximal plaster is trimmed with a Le Cron carver, and the die gently pushed out of the master cast in the manner described above. After removal of the die the proximal areas of the die housing are further trimmed to allow room for a platinum matrix (Chapter 5).

One disadvantage of the technique so far described is that tapering or ill-defined preparations are difficult to position in the localizing impression and this can result in the restoration being back to front, the contacts being too loose or too tight, or the occlusion being too high. To avoid these problems, many operators modify the above technique, as described below, to give a more positive localization of the die.

Modified technique

When preparing the copper ring at the chairside the dental surgeon cuts a 4 mm long 'V' at the incisal end. The impression is taken in the normal way and, whilst the impression is *in situ*, the excess

Fig. 1.10 To remove the die of a porcelain jacket crown from a master cast the plaster around the neck of the die is removed.

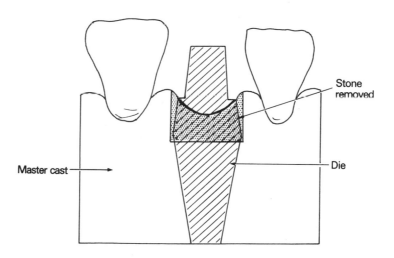

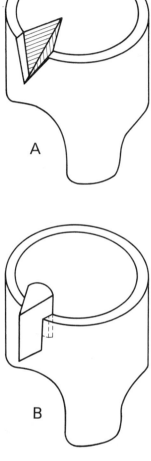

Fig. 1.11 Localizing devices. (A) The copper ring and compound are prepared by cutting a 'V' notch into the incisal end of the ring and impression compound. (B) A plastic localizing rod may be used.

compound is removed from around the outside of the copper ring. At the same time a V-shaped piece of compound is removed through the cut in the ring (Fig. 1.11). Alternatively a plastic localizing rod (see Appendix) is positioned on the incisal end of the ring (Fig. 1.11). With the impression still *in situ* an alginate localizing impression is taken. When the impression is removed from the mouth a V-shaped extension will be visible in the alginate which is used later to localize the die.

1   As before, copper is deposited upon the impression, backed with acrylic resin and a dowel pin inserted.

2   At this point the technique varies slightly. The die is left in the compound impression and the excess resin trimmed to a smooth finish with the sides of the copper ring. The die and copper ring are lubricated and, using the 'V' notch or plastic rod, the die is localized in the alginate impression, which is boxed with carding wax, the die supported by a traversing wire and the cast poured.

3   When the master cast has set, the sides of the ring are carefully cleared of plaster, to prevent the ring damaging the adjacent teeth, and the die removed.

4   The compound impression is then removed from the die which is trimmed as before.

Casts from a rubber base impression

It is generally accepted that rubber base is not the easiest material to use, the technique being a little messy and requiring some form of gingival retraction to obtain an impression of subgingival margins, but these problems are outweighed by the technical advantages. The cast is accurate, more than one cast can be poured in the impression, the construction of the cast is quick and easy and the necessity to localize dies is eliminated, which make it ideal for multiple restorations.

Special tray

Although rubber base is costly compared with other impression materials, the cost of rubber base impressions can be minimized by the use of a closely-adapted tray, specially made for each patient. Special trays also produce an even thickness of material throughout the impression which reduces the likelihood of distortion. To be efficient a special tray should be rigid, an autopolymerizing acrylic resin being an ideal material in this respect. It is constructed upon the study cast in the following way.

1   Five dental napkins are folded to give ten layers, moistened, and excess water wrung out. These are laid and closely adapted over the coronal area of the cast. There is no need to cover the palate since in most cases the teeth only are involved in the restorative programme. Taking an impression of the palate would waste impression material and cause unnecessary discomfort to the patient. Alternatively, it is possible to use asbestos strip as a spacer. The use of wax as a spacer is to be deprecated because polymerization of acrylic resin produces an exothermic reaction resulting in the wax melting and becoming messy to remove from the cast and the inside of the tray.

2   Autopolymerizing acrylic resins are available for construction of closely adapted trays. The material is mixed to a dough consistency as recommended by the manufacturer and rolled into a cylinder about 13 mm in diameter. A piece approximately 26 mm long is cut off and replaced in the mixing pot. The remainder is flattened until it is about 2 mm thick and long enough to stretch from the distal edge of the last tooth on one side of the cast along the occlusal table to the distal edge of the last tooth on the other side. It is then adapted closely to the buccal, occlusal and lingual surfaces of the cast and extended 2–3 mm beyond the gingival margins of the crowns.

3   A handle is formed from the material left in the mixing pot. It is flattened to form a ribbon about 32 mm long, 19 mm wide and 2 mm thick. A little monomer is placed in the mixing pot and the end of the ribbon moistened in it. The ribbon is then held in the vertical position and pressed onto the tray in the incisor region. There is usually a little resin left adhering to the sides of the pot; with the aid of the monomer this is scraped onto a spatula and used to attach the handle to the tray. The first 10 mm of the handle are then left vertical whilst the remainder is bent horizontally (Fig. 1.12) and supported until polymerization is complete. This allows the handle to rise over the lip when placed in the mouth.

4   When polymerization is complete, the napkins are removed from

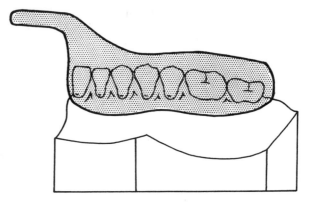

Fig. 1.12 A closely-adapted tray should extend only 2–3 mm beyond the gingival areas. The handle must rise over the lip.

the tray which is then trimmed on a grinding wheel to finish the periphery 2–3 mm beyond the gingival margins of the teeth. It is unnecessary to extend such a tray well into the buccal sulcus in the manner required for dentures. The tray is smoothed using an acrylic trimmer, finally finishing with sandpaper. Three occlusal stops may be incorporated in the tray to prevent it being inadvertently forced onto the prepared teeth. These stops are small additions of wax or autopolymerizing resin (1 mm thick × 2 mm wide × 5 mm long) placed on the occlusal inner surface of the tray. One stop is placed over an unprepared posterior tooth on each side of the arch and one over an unprepared anterior tooth. It is then ready for use in the surgery at the patient's second visit.

Die stone cast

After the dentist has taken a rubber base impression it is necessary to allow 15–30 minutes to elapse before a cast is poured into it. This allows the elastic memory of the material to eliminate distortion caused by removing the impression from the mouth. Casts may be poured up to 48 hours after taking the impression and are still sufficiently accurate, but after this period distortions occur which become evident when the restorations are tried in the mouth.

Pouring the cast

1   The impression is checked for blood and saliva, any present being washed and gently brushed off. The impression is then dried, using a dental napkin.

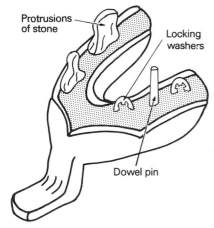

Fig. 1.13 Stone around the base of the die should be perfectly smooth. Retention, in the form of locking washers or well-roughened protrusions of die stone, is placed either side of the dowel pin and at random throughout the rest of the dentition.

2 To help with positioning the dowel pin at a later stage the centre of the coronal area of the prepared tooth is marked with a ball point pen on the sides of the impression.

3 The die stone is mixed to a putty consistency (30 g powder to 7 ml water) which gives a working time of 5 minutes. Starting at the heels, the stone is carefully and slowly vibrated along the floor of the impression until it is about 3 mm above the gingival margin of the teeth. The stone around the base of the die should be perfectly smooth. Retention, in the form of locking washers or well-roughened protrusions of die stone, is placed on both sides of the die and at random throughout the rest of the dentition (Fig. 1.13) to attach it to the basing-off plaster.

4 The die is completed by using the pen marks (see **2**, above) on the sides of the impression to position the knurled end of a Universal dowel pin (or its equivalent) into the die stone.

5 When the die stone has set, after approximately 20 minutes, a large round bur, size 10–12, is used to make a depression in the stone 3 mm either labially or lingually to the dowel pin. This acts as an antirotational device preventing movement of the die. A thin machine oil is used to lightly lubricate the pin and the surrounding die stone at its base, and a small ball of carding wax placed on the apex of the dowel pin to help locate it after basing off with plaster.

6 A mixture of equal parts of plaster and Kaffir 'D' is vibrated onto the base of the die stone. The remainder is placed in a plastic disposable base former and the impression inverted onto it. Alternatively, the impression may be boxed with carding wax and the plaster–Kaffir 'D' mix poured into it.

7 No attempt should be made to remove the impression from the cast until 1 hour after casting the die stone.

8 To remove the impression from the cast, the excess plaster is first removed from the tray. The handle is then firmly held and pulled in an occlusal direction. A rocking motion should not be used because this could result in a fractured die.

Alternative method
An alternative way is to incorporate metal strips in the impression. These are placed over the margins where they help to shape the die and delineate its base for positioning the dowel pin.

Die stone hardeners. A better working surface can be formed on the die by coating it with a solution of 10% polystyrene in amyl acetate. This is painted onto the surface of the die, the excess blown off, and then allowed to dry for about 5 minutes. Mineral oils may also be used (see Appendix).

ARTICULATING

An occlusal registration is not generally required when constructing the single restoration if full-mouth upper and lower impressions are taken. When extensive restorative measures are undertaken wax or zinc oxide paste occlusal records or wax registration blocks are advisable to ensure accurate mounting of the casts on an articulator.

Articulators may have a simple hinge movement, a fixed condylar path or an adjustable condylar path. It is generally accepted that the adjustable condylar path articulator is superior to all others as far as prosthetic dentistry is concerned, and there are

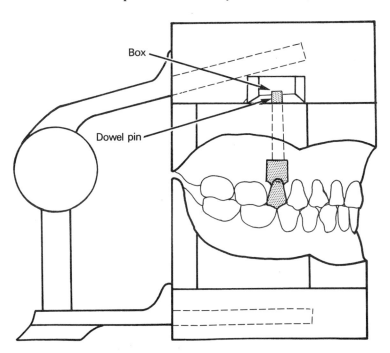

Fig. 1.16 When articulating, an open box is formed over the apex of the dowel pin to allow access.

many who feel the same applies to restorative dentistry. It is often found, however, that where the full dentition is concerned it is not always possible to reproduce the patient's mandibular movements even on an adjustable articulator, with the result that cuspal locking still occurs. There is no doubt that in all cases of full mouth rehabilitation the fully adjustable articulator should be used but, for the single restoration and small bridges, the simple hinge articulator is satisfactory. Descriptions of these articulators are available in books on prosthetic dentistry, so only the slight variation on mounting the cast will be described here.

When articulating casts it must be remembered that there are dies present which must be removed during the construction of the restoration, so access to the apex of the die must be allowed. This is accomplished by forming an open box over the apex of the dowel pin on the exterior border of the base of the cast. It is formed by a block of wax being placed over the dowel pin. If the casts are mounted on the articulator in the normal manner, and then the wax removed, a space will have been left over the dowel pin (Fig. 1.16). An instrument may then be inserted to remove the die from the cast.

2   The Pattern

Having poured and articulated the casts a pattern (or precursor of the restoration) is made on the die in wax. This is embedded in a refractory material which is heated to burn out the wax, thus leaving a space or mould into which molten metal is poured to form the restoration. Though more accurate nowadays, this is still basically the same 'lost wax process' used by the ancient Egyptians. A pattern may thus be formed to fit any cavity or tooth specially prepared to accept a metal casting. The formation of patterns to fit the following preparations will be described: inlay, veneer crown, pin inlay (pinlay) and intraradicular post.

Instruments.   The instruments which are found useful when making a wax pattern are a Le Cron carver, Ash No. 5, a small wax knife and a small paint brush (No. 3). A piece of dental gauze for wiping wax off the instruments, and a pledget of cotton wool for polishing the finished wax pattern, are also convenient.

It is advisable for the production of smooth patterns to have the blade of the Le Cron carver highly polished.

Separating mediums.   Wax will stick to the surface of the die unless the die is coated with a separating medium, so detergents such as Teepol are used. Separators should be used sparingly since puddles on the surface of a die give an inaccurate fitting surface to the wax pattern. An acceptable method of application is to use a paint brush, the excess liquid being blown off to prevent bubbling of the medium.

Inlays are constructed to fit every type of cavity from Class I to V. They may have buccal or lingual extensions, and they may be extended onto the tops of cusps to form capped cusps. No matter which type of inlay is made, the method of construction is the same.

They are all formed first in inlay wax. This is supplied as sticks

18

which are softened over a Bunsen burner flame, in warm water, or in a warm oven. Although many operators believe there is less likelihood of burning out the constituents when using the second and third methods, the first method is probably the most widely used.

When using the Bunsen burner method, the wax is held high above the flame to soften it without melting, and is intermittently kneaded gently with the fingers to produce a uniform softness throughout the mass. It is essential to keep the manipulative temperature of these waxes as near as possible to room temperature because, if overheated, constituents will burn out resulting in a deterioration of the physical properties of the wax. Wax expands when heated and contracts upon cooling, but since the contraction never equals expansion, stresses result within the wax. By reducing the manipulative temperature, the degree of stress is reduced. Pressure exerted as the wax solidifies can also reduce the inherent stresses.

Wax is adapted to a die by pressing softened wax onto the die with the fingers until it has solidified, or by pouring molten wax onto the die, followed by finger pressure until it has hardened. It is generally accepted that more accurate inlays are produced by the first method.

PATTERN FOR INLAYS

1 After lubrication of the die, inlay wax is carefully softened over a Bunsen burner flame and intermittently kneaded between the fingers to produce an homogeneous soft mass. When completely soft, it is adapted to the die with index finger and thumb and held until the wax solidifies. The excess wax at the margins and cusps is removed with a warm Le Cron carver. Upon removing the pattern from the die the fitting surface is examined; the line angles and margins should be sharp and well-defined—if they are not, another pattern should be formed. When the fitting surface is satisfactory the die is relubricated and the pattern repositioned.

2 It should be remembered that the proximal contact area of posterior teeth lies within the buccal half of the tooth, with the lingual aspect of the tooth narrower than the buccal (Fig. 2.1).

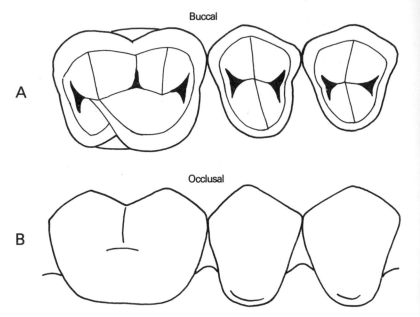

Fig. 2.1 (A) The contact area of the posterior teeth lies within the buccal half of the tooth, with the lingual aspect of the tooth narrower than the buccal. (B) The embrasures are formed by the proximal surfaces of the teeth and the positioning of the marginal ridges.

Correct contact area positions are important because they prevent food from being packed into the interdental papillae, which could lead to caries, destruction of the gingiva and damage to the periodontal membranes. Contact areas also stabilize the teeth within the dental arch. The contacts are checked, molten wax being added to form a snug fit with the adjacent tooth.

3   The embrasures are also important and are formed by the proximal surfaces of the teeth and the positioning of the marginal ridge (Fig. 2.1). Embrasures perform three functions: they act as spillways during mastication, allowing the bolus of food to flow off the occlusal table to prevent a build up of excessive forces on the teeth; they allow stimulation of the tissues by food, tongue and cheeks; and they allow the teeth to be cleaned easily.

4   If a warm Le Cron carver is used like a butter knife, the carver will adapt the wax to the margins and at the same time remove the excess. Patterns should be a perfect fit and finish exactly at the margins because over-extended margins may lead to oral disease.

5   Although the occlusal surface can be carved by using a cold Le Cron carver, smoother patterns may be obtained by using a warm

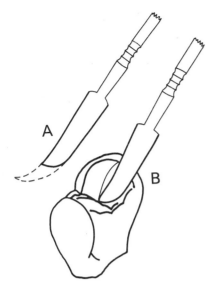

Fig. 2.2 The point of the blade of the Le Cron carver should be rounded (A) when it then resembles the facet of a cusp (B).

one. The point of a Le Cron carver is too sharp for the latter technique, and the instrument may be adapted by rounding off the point of the blade and highly polishing the trimmed end, so that the end of the blade resembles the side of a cusp (Fig. 2.2). If the blade is gently heated and then lightly pressed onto the occlusal surface of a pattern the marginal ridge will be formed, and so will the side of the cusp, and it will be found that the occlusal surface may be formed in a very few minutes. The contours of the remaining cusps of the natural dentition are followed and, where possible, the cuspal angle and the depth of the fissures are reduced. The further back in the mouth the tooth is the less the cuspal angle should be. Shallow carving enables the finished casting to be polished more easily, reduces the occlusal load on the tooth and decreases the risk of cheek biting.

6   The marginal ridge should be at the same height as, and the same width as, the marginal ridge of the adjacent tooth. If placed too close to the centre of the tooth, a proximal incline plane will be produced, down which food will slide and cause food packing, to the detriment of the periodontal tissues and the frequent annoyance of the patient. The occlusion is checked against the opposing cast throughout the procedure. Overcontouring of the occlusal surface may cause a great deal of inconvenience to the dentist, involving grinding and repolishing of the inlay prior to fitting.

7   When contouring has been completed, the surface of the wax is smoothed by soaking a pledget of cotton wool in a degreasing agent (Teepol), warming it over a Bunsen flame and rubbing it over the wax. It should be remembered that a rough pattern will never produce a smooth casting.

VENEER CROWNS

It is necessary to make veneer crowns for some patients. The first step in preparation of this type of restoration is the reduction of the outer surface of the tooth by an even thickness of tissue. The restoration formed to fit over such a preparation is called a veneer crown and may be a full veneer crown (shell crown) with the restoration covering the whole of the crown, or a partial veneer crown (three-quarter crown) with the labial or buccal surface of the crown excluded from the restoration. Full veneers may be constructed entirely in metal, or in a combination of metal with either acrylic resin or porcelain on the labial surface. The simplest type of full veneer crown is the 'thimble'.

Thimble

A thimble is a thin metal veneer placed over a full veneer preparation to improve the shape, to increase its height, to produce a shoulder on a fractured incisor when an oblique fracture has involved the root, or to form a labial shoulder on lower anteriors. The thimble may be used as a retainer in bridge work (see Chapter 4) when a proximal shoulder is produced for soldering purposes, or to straighten the alignment of preparations which would otherwise be impossible to align and is then one part of a telescopic crown.

The thimble is formed in sheet casting wax with inlay wax added to produce the required shape, the technique being the basis for the construction of all veneer crowns. The thickness of the sheet wax is varied from 0·2–0·4 mm according to the amount of tooth tissue removed.

1 The die is lubricated and a strip of sheet casting wax is closely adapted to it forming a butt joint where the two ends meet and carefully sealing them with inlay wax.

2 The shape of the thimble is adjusted with inlay wax to produce the required contour, and the pattern smoothed (Fig. 2.3).

Full veneer crown

1 After adapting a piece of sheet casting wax to the die and sealing the join with inlay wax, the excess at the gingival margin is removed by sweeping a Le Cron carver blade around the groove cut into the die (Chapter 1). Excess wax extending above the occlusal surface is also removed.

2 A further piece of sheet wax is adapted to the occlusal surface and sealed to the collar to form a cap (Fig. 2.4), which is then

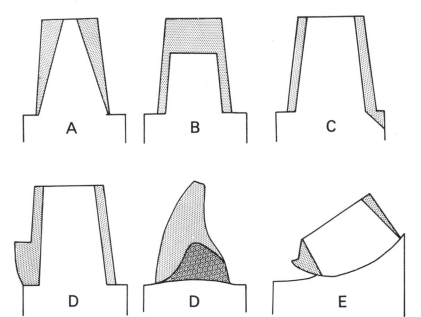

Fig. 2.3 Types of thimble: (A) producing increased retention form; (B) increasing the height of the preparation; (C) producing a shoulder when an oblique fracture of the crown has involved the root; (D) producing a proximal shoulder when the tooth is to be used as a retainer in bridge work; (E) telescopic crown used to align a preparation in bridge work.

removed and the fitting surface examined to ensure it is crease free. The die is relubricated and the wax cap reseated.

(The next stage is to build the crown to the required anatomical form by dripping wax onto the cap. This needs skilful handling of the Le Cron carver and inlay wax, the handle end of the blade being heated rather than the tip because wax runs away from the source of heat; the wax therefore remains at the tip where it is required. The carver is used like a fibretip pen, the operator visualizing colouring the crown with blue ink.)

3   A little inlay wax is melted on the end of the Le Cron carver, the edge of the globule of wax placed against the sheet wax and the shape of the cusp drawn. More wax is used to shape the cusp along the bucco-occlusal angle; then the centre of the cusp is filled (Fig. 2.4). During this stage the upper and lower casts are occluded, the wax being added until the cusp contacts the opposing dentition. Each cusp is built in this manner (Fig. 2.4).

4   The mesiolingual cusp of the upper first and second molars needs special mention (Fig. 2.5). Starting at the mesiobuccal angle of the buccal triangular cusp the marginal ridge is outlined; then by

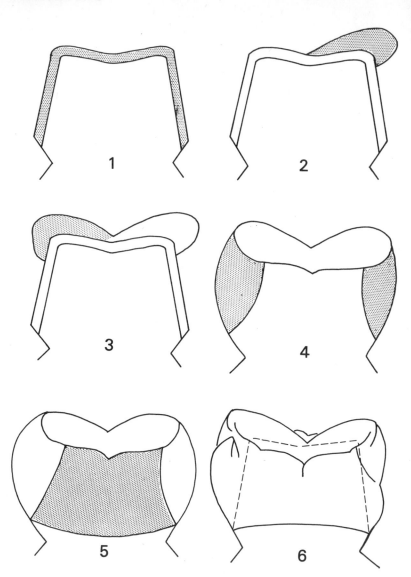

Fig. 2.4 Stages of construction of a full veneer crown. (1) Wax cap. (2) The cusp is formed using inlay wax. Note how it overhangs the bucco-occlusal angle. (3) All the cusps are formed in the same manner. (4) Buccal and lingual walls built. (5) Proximal surfaces flushed with inlay wax. (6) The crown is contoured to the required shape using a warm Le Cron carver.

curving the wax onto the lingual-occlusal angle the mesiolingual cusp is outlined until the centre of the tooth is reached, when it sweeps obliquely across the occlusal surface to meet the apex of the distobuccal cusp. The procedure is repeated until the cusp is well defined; then the centre of the cusp is filled and the casts occluded.

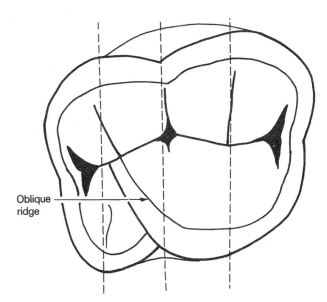

Oblique ridge

Fig. 2.5 Upper first molar. The oblique ridge starts to traverse the occlusal surface half way along the occlusolingual angle.

5 The outer walls of the tooth are formed in the same manner. The shape of the cusp is outlined and the centre filled with wax until the required contour is obtained. A little wax flushed along the proximal surfaces forms the contact areas and the proximal embrasures, and joins the buccal and lingual cusps. These are checked by placing the die in the master cast. Wax is flushed between the cusps to produce an even curvature.

6 The final occlusal contouring is accomplished by the use of a warm Le Cron carver as suggested for inlay construction.

The contour of the buccal and lingual walls is important because the middle and cervical thirds of the crown are responsible for deflecting food over the gingival margin to stimulate the tissues in this area. Undercontouring can lead to food packing whilst overcontouring produces stagnation areas. The curvature of the natural crown extends over the gingiva by 0·5–1·0 mm (Fig. 2.6). An Ash No. 5 wax carver is a useful instrument for shaping these surfaces. The full veneer crown is the most difficult restoration to contour, the replacement of the large amount of tissue removed requiring a full knowledge and understanding of tooth morphology.

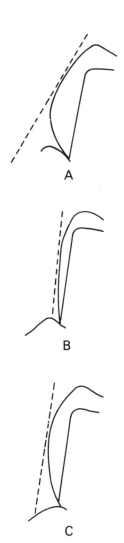

Fig. 2.6 (A) Overcontouring of a crown can produce stagnation areas. (B) Undercontouring results in food packing into the gingival crevice. (C) The curvature of the natural crown extends over the gingival margin by 0·5–1·0 mm.

Partial veneer crown

1 A wax cap is adapted to the lubricated die and the ends sealed on the buccal surface.

2 A little inlay wax is melted on a Le Cron carver and starting at the end of one groove the sheet wax is penetrated to deposit inlay wax along the entire length of all the grooves. Pressure is exerted on the wax as it solidifies to obtain a perfect impression of the grooves.

3 Excess wax is removed from the buccal surface to finish the pattern at the proximal margins and the fitting surface examined for the presence of well-defined grooves. The die is relubricated and the pattern repositioned in readiness to contour the crown in the manner described for full veneer crowns.

4 The labio-incisal or bucco-occlusal wax edge should be kept inconspicuous by carefully rounding it towards the lingual surface and keeping it as thin as possible.

PINLAY AND PINLEDGE

1 After adapting sheet wax to the die, the pin holes and ledges are exposed by removing a little wax in these areas.

2 Pins are inserted into the holes and molten wax dripped around the pin heads and onto the ledges (see Appendix). The fragility of this pattern prevents examination of the fitting surface until the contour of the pattern has been completed in the manner described above (Fig. 2.7).

INTRARADICULAR POSTS

An intraradicular post accurately fits the prepared root canal of a tooth requiring the restoration of the whole of its crown. These are called post crowns. There are two types of post, the preformed commercially produced ones such as Charlton, Kurer, Mooser, etc, and the laboratory cast type. The relative merits of the commercially produced posts over laboratory prepared posts is beyond the scope

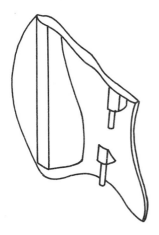

Fig. 2.7 Pinledge.

of this book, but with each type the crown is restored by an acrylic or porcelain jacket crown (Chapters 5 and 7) or by a bonded porcelain crown (Chapter 6). All such crowns are cemented to a coronal extension of the post so that should the crown ever need renewal the post can remain undisturbed in the root canal.

Only the laboratory-produced post will be described, the most common being the 'cast post and core'. The post is individually made to fit the patient's prepared root canal accurately with the coronal extension built to the shape of a porcelain jacket crown preparation. The post is formed in wax before the core, but they are cast as an integral unit.

1 A length of plastic rod (a plastic dowel pin is ideal) is trimmed to a loose fit inside the root canal of the die and its surface flushed with inlay wax. This is inserted, whilst the wax is soft, into the lubricated root canal and held firmly until the wax solidifies. It is then removed and examined; the wax should be smooth and even—if it is not the process is repeated. Occasionally, when a die has been constructed from a rubber base impression, an undercut is present within the root canal. In such cases the waxed rod is pushed in and out of the canal a few times to drag the wax out of the undercut before it solidifies.

2 The rod is carefully sawn through so that about 1 mm of the post protrudes above the root face (Fig. 2.8). After relubrication of the die, the post is replaced.

3 To form the core, molten wax is added to the top of the post until it is almost the full width of the root face and two-thirds of the original height of the crown. This is contoured in accordance with the following principles (Fig. 2.8):

   a The contour of the core is kept within the general contour of the natural crown.

   b An even shoulder, normally 1 mm wide, should be formed around the root face.

   c The proximal surfaces should be parallel in the vertical plane and palatally inclined in the horizontal plane.

   d The cingulum area should be nearly parallel with the labial surface.

   e The incisal third of the labial surface should have a lingual curve.

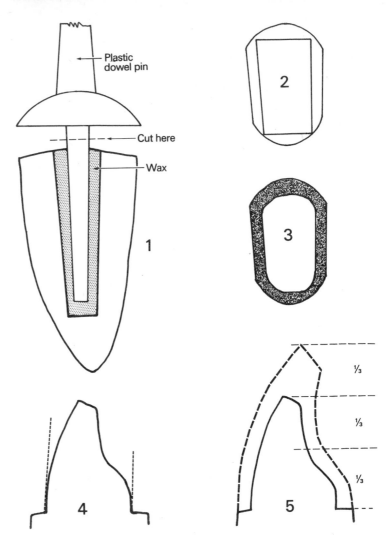

Fig. 2.8 Construction of a cast post and core. (1) Constructing the post. (2) The proximal surfaces of the core should be palatally inclined in the horizontal plane. (3) All line angles should be rounded off. (4) The cingulum area should be nearly parallel with the labial surface. (5) The core should be two-thirds the length of the original crown.

f   The core should be two-thirds the length of the original crown.
g   All angles should be gently rounded.

A slightly warmed scalpel is ideal for shaping the core, which should allow sufficient clearance for the crown: this is determined by occluding the casts.

Alternative method

Another method is to form the core inside an alumina tube—it is then referred to as a spigot.

1   The post is formed in the manner described above.

2   An oval alumina tube of suitable size is selected, cut to the required length and one end countersunk.

3   The next stage is the formation of a wax rod to fit snugly into the tube. A wax sprue former made of metal is filled with sheet casting wax, then warmed over a Bunsen burner flame. An alumina tube the same size as that to be used in the restoration is lubricated and held over the largest hole of the sprue former so that wax extrudes through it (Fig. 2.9). The wax expands as it is extruded, therefore, after extrusion, the tube is relubricated and the wax rod gently pushed through the tube again until it is a snug fit. The wax rod is cut to double the length of the alumina tube and inserted into it.

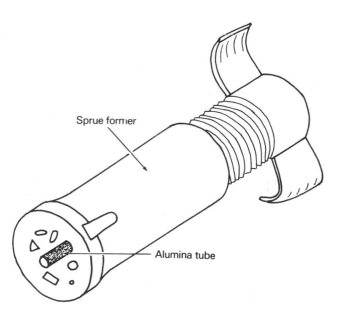

Sprue former

Alumina tube

Fig. 2.9   Metal former for making wax sprues. The alumina tube is held against the widest hole on the base of the sprue former.

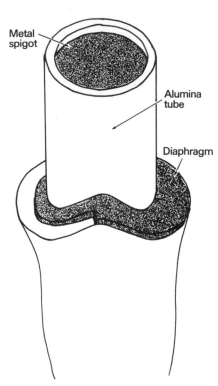

Metal spigot

Alumina tube

Diaphragm

Fig. 2.10   Preparation of an alumina tube post crown.

4   The alumina tube is then positioned, counter-sunk end towards the post, at the required angle and the spigot waxed to the post (Fig. 2.10). A wax diaphragm may be added to the lingual aspect of the tooth to form a shoulder or to accommodate proximal connectors in bridge work (Chapter 4). The tube is removed from the spigot, and a sprue former attached.

SPRUEING

For molten metal to be poured into a mould there must be a passage through the refractory material to the mould. The most satisfactory method is to form this passage at the time of embedding the pattern. This is done by attaching rods of wax and/or metal, called sprue formers, to the pattern.

Point of attachment

The walls of the mould can assist or impede the flow of the metal as it enters the mould, depending upon the positioning of the sprue former. For example, when a sprue former is attached to the side of a V-shaped inlay, such as a mesio-occlusal inlay (M.O.) the metal hits the flat wall of the mould and rebounds causing turbulence which slows the flow of metal (Fig. 2.11). By attaching a sprue former to the point of the V the walls of the mould assist flow of the metal, ensuring rapid filling of the mould (Fig. 2.11).

Diameter

The thinnest sections of a casting are the first to cool and contract, drawing upon the molten metal in the thicker sections, but the thicker sections must also have a reservoir of molten metal upon which to draw. Sprues can act as ideal reservoirs if attached to the thickest sections of the casting and should be at least as thick as the thickest part of the pattern. Failure to do this invariably produces pits throughout the casting, called porosity.

If it is difficult to attach a thick sprue former to a pattern a thin one may be used provided it is thickened to form a reservoir close to the casting and no further than 2 mm from the pattern (Fig.

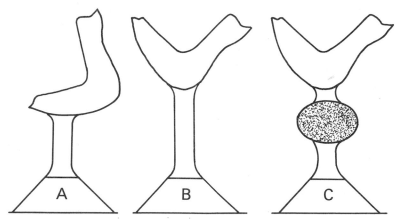

Fig. 2.11 Sprue attachment: (A) incorrectly attached; (B) correctly attached; (C) position of a reservoir.

2.11). The thickest areas, and the easiest from which to remove the sprue after casting, are the tips of cusps and marginal ridges.

Length

Every mould contains gases which must be expelled as the metal enters, otherwise they prevent the mould from being completely

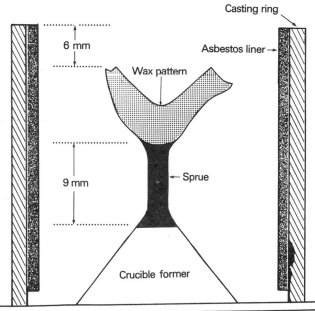

Fig. 2.12 Wax pattern positioned inside the casting cylinder.

filled. Four factors govern the rate of gas expulsion: the permeability of the refractory material; the thickness of the refractory material between the top of the pattern and the top of the casting ring (the back-up investment); the length of the sprue hole; and the presence of air vents around the mould (see Chapter 3). Experience has shown that the back-up investment should be no thicker than 6 mm and the sprue former 9 mm long (Fig. 2.12). The use of air vents depends upon the permeability of the refractory material being used (see Chapter 3).

The patterns described are sprued as shown in Fig. 2.13.

Attaching the sprue

The first sprue attached should be metal to support the pattern; the others can be wax, but they must all be kept to the same length. The

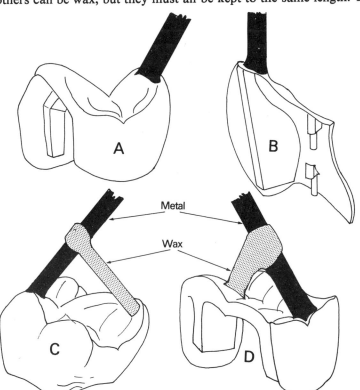

Fig. 2.13 Recommended sprue positions for various patterns. (A) Partial veneer crown. (B) Pinledge. (C) Full veneer crown. (D) Mesio-occluso-distal inlay (M.O.D.).

end of the metal sprue former is warmed in a Bunsen burner flame and placed on the surface of the pattern, where it is held steady until the melted wax solidifies, the point of attachment of the sprue former being slightly flared with wax. The wax sprue former is held over the point of attachment and sealed to the pattern with a lightly warmed Le Cron carver. It is then firmly sealed to the metal sprue former by wax, which is run completely around the metal.

Sprueing substructures (see Chapter 6)

The alloys used to construct substructures for bonded porcelain crowns are more viscous at casting temperatures than normal gold alloys so thicker sprues are needed, the minimum thickness being 2 mm. A porosity-free casting is essential because porous metal releases gases during the bonding process seriously affecting the efficiency of the bond. Some manufacturers recommend that the sprue former should be narrower at the point of attachment. A variation is the use of short sprue formers about 7 mm long attached to a horizontal 4 mm thick bar, which is attached in turn to primary sprues terminating at the crucible former, (Fig. 2.14) this method being said to produce the most dense casting. Large reservoirs are recommended when the conventional method of sprueing is used.

Annealing the pattern

Thin patterns, such as thimbles and substructures for bonded porcelain work, often warp. This tendency may be minimized by placing the sprued pattern, still on the master cast, in a thermostatically controlled water bath for 10 minutes at a setting of 30°C.

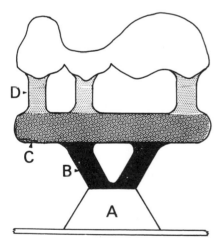

Fig. 2.14 Alternative sprueing technique for bridge work. (A) Crucible former. (B) Primary sprues. (C) Horizontal bar reservoir. (D) Individual sprues.

DIRECT PATTERNS

So far consideration has been given to indirect patterns. The procedures to be followed for direct patterns is similar but they are often sprued in the mouth, which can be difficult especially when the pattern is positioned distally in a posterior tooth. In such a case the dental surgeon usually removes the pattern on the end of a probe and

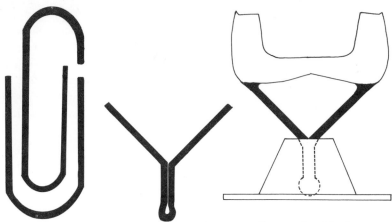

Fig. 2.15 Sprueing an M.O.D. pattern using a paper clip.

sprues it out of the mouth. Metal paper clips make ideal sprue formers when sprueing in the mouth, especially for the Mesio-occlusal-distal inlay (M.O.D.) when the clip is bent as shown in Fig. 2.15. It is essential to keep the bend in the wire outside the refractory material to permit removal.

Discrepancies in the pattern may be adjusted by the use of low melting-point wax, such as carding wax. Any blood and saliva on the pattern is removed by washing it in a solution of equal parts of soft soap and hydrogen peroxide, then washing in water. Traces of cavity lining should also be removed before investing.

CRUCIBLE FORMERS

It would be difficult to pour molten metal down a small sprue hole, so a funnel should also be formed in the refractory material. This is done by using a cone-shaped piece of metal called a crucible former (Fig. 2.12). The top of the former is usually flat when new, but it may be beaten into a dome shape before use and a hole drilled through its centre to allow fixing of the sprue former.

The former is greased lightly to prevent refractory material adhering to it. The sprued pattern is carefully removed from the die and the sprue former inserted into the hole in the crucible former, its length being adjusted to 9 mm before it is waxed to the crucible former (Fig. 2.12). The pattern is then ready for covering with the refractory investment material, this procedure being called 'investing'.

3   Investing, Casting and Finishing Procedures

When the pattern has been formed, sprued and attached to a crucible former it is enclosed in a cylinder which is then filled with a refractory based material called investment, the technique being known as investing. The investment is heated, thus eliminating the wax to form the mould into which metal is poured, this process being called casting. The casting is finished by removal of surface oxides and polishing. The physical properties of a casting may be modified by controlled heating and cooling, known as heat treatment.

INVESTING

Ideally, investment materials should produce sufficient expansion to compensate for shrinkage of the metal, be capable of reproducing fine detail, and withstand high temperatures and casting forces without distortion or cracking when metal is thrust into the mould. They should be sufficiently permeable to allow mould gases to escape yet produce a smooth mould surface, and set within 15–30 minutes. Finally, they should be easily removable from the casting.

There are basically three types of investment which contain silicon dioxide in the form of quartz, tridymite or crystobalite as the main constituent and refractory material. The particles are bound by gypsum, silicate (ethyl or sodium) or phosphate (ammonium diacid phosphate), the investment being named after the binder used. When gypsum-bonded investments are heated in a furnace above 700°C in the presence of carbon (wax deposits) they start to decompose, so this limits their use to the lower fusing alloys. Higher fusing alloys are cast into the silicate- or phosphate-bonded investments. Investing procedures are the same for all.

Preparing the cylinder

1   A metal cylinder 30 mm by 40 mm is lined with an asbestos strip 1 mm thick and 5 mm shorter than the height of the cylinder. It is moistened with water and adapted to the inside of the cylinder, with one edge flush with the end of the cylinder. This allows investment to grip the cylinder at the other end.

2   The cylinder is placed over the pattern, exposed end against the crucible former and the sprue former length adjusted to bring the pattern 6 mm from the top (Fig. 2.12). It is then sealed to the crucible former with wax.

Air vents

Silicate- and phosphate-bonded investments are less permeable to mould gases than those bonded with gypsum, so air vents or breathers are placed around the pattern to help dissipate the gases (Fig. 3.1). When gypsum-bonded investments are used, air vents are also positioned around full veneer patterns.

A length of No. 2 wax sprue former is bent into the shape of a letter L and attached to the top of the cylinder with one end inside the concavity of the full veneer pattern, the other end being firmly sealed to the cylinder to prevent displacement during investing (Fig. 3.1). It is essential that the vent is not allowed to touch the pattern, otherwise metal would be lost through the vent during casting.

Investing in air

1   Investment is mixed according to the manufacturer's instructions and vibrated to eliminate trapped air.

2   The cylinder and crucible former are held with the thumb on the top edge of the cylinder and the fingers supporting the crucible former. The backs of the supporting fingers are rested on the vibrator and a little investment vibrated down the inside surface of the cylinder. As the cylinder fills, it is rocked from side to side to dislodge trapped air which, if not eliminated, causes rough castings

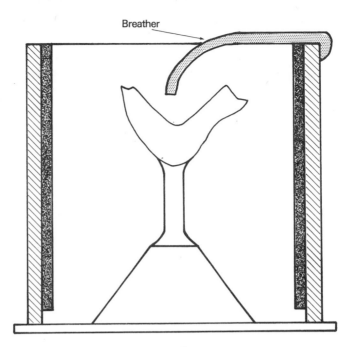

Breather

Fig. 3.1 Positioning of an air vent or breather.

involving lengthy finishing procedures. Vibration is continued until the cylinder has been filled completely when it is placed on a surface away from the vibrator.

3 Silicate- and phosphate-bonded investments are thicker than gypsum-bonded ones, therefore air inclusions are more difficult to avoid. These may be minimized by painting the pattern with a precoating medium of ammonia and fine silica particles, before being covered with a casting cylinder.

4 All investments are allowed to set for 30–60 minutes before proceeding to the heating and casting stage.

Vacuum investing

Vacuum investing assists in elimination of air inclusions. There are many expensive commercial vacuum-investing machines, all basically consisting of a vacuum motor, mechanical spatulator and vibrator. The technique is generally explained in detail in the

manufacturer's instruction booklet, so this will not be described
here. Instead a simple vacuum invester designed by Morrant and
modified by Allan and Moore is described (Fig. 3.2; see Appendix).

The apparatus consists of a bottle with a rubber cap, through
which passes a glass or metal tube onto which is attached a rubber
tube.

1 The tubing and valve are attached to the water tap, the water
turned on and a check made to ensure that there is no blockage, by
feeling for suction at the end of the tube. The water is turned off, the
tube attached to the bottle and the open end of a casting cylinder
placed into the rubber cap.

2 Investment is mixed in a rubber bowl and vibrated into the
bottle, after which the rubber cap is assembled on the bottle and a
vacuum created. Keeping the tube uppermost the bottle is slowly
tipped and the investment vibrated into the casting cylinder until this
has been filled.

3 It is essential to clean the vacuum apparatus immediately after
use since hardened investment is difficult to remove from a glass
container, and cleanliness assists the production of a vacuum.

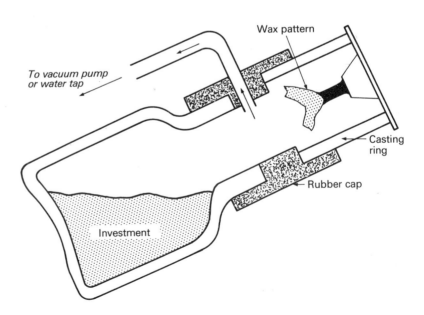

Fig. 3.2 The Allan and Moore
vacuum investing bottle.

CASTING

To compensate for the contraction of metal on cooling it is important that sufficient expansion is developed in the mould. This is accomplished by setting expansion, hygroscopic expansion, and by thermal or inversion expansion (see Appendix).

Setting expansion takes place immediately the pattern has been invested, the maximum being reached in the first 12 hours and reducing over the next 12 hours. An increased setting expansion (*hygroscopic expansion*) can be obtained in gypsum-bonded investments by the addition of water to the setting mixture.

To obtain the maximum benefit from these two methods the metal should be cast into the mould between 6 and 12 hours after investing. *Thermal* or *inversion expansion* takes place when the investment is heated in a furnace, due mainly to the silica inverting from its alpha to its beta form.

The crucible former and metal sprue former are removed before heating the investment.

1 The crucible former is warmed and then held in one hand and the casting cylinder in the other. A careful twisting motion of the hands in opposite directions pulls the crucible away from the cylinder. Dislodged investment falls away or is brushed or blown off.

2 The casting cylinder is held over a Bunsen burner with the sprue former downwards in the flame until warm. The sprue former should be kept inverted so that when it is gripped with a pair of pliers and carefully withdrawn from the investment by a to-and-fro twisting movement, dislodged investment will fall away from the sprue hole and not down it. Loose investment at the mouth of the mould is removed.

3 Gypsum-bonded investment is heated by angling the cylinder against an inside wall of a cold furnace and the temperature raised to 700°C. Alternatively the cylinder is placed in a preheating oven, the temperature of which is raised to 400°C, then the cylinder transferred to a furnace which has been preheated to 700°C. If silicate- or phosphate-bonded investments are used the cylinder is heated to 850°C when precious metal-based alloys are to be cast into them, or to 960°C when chrome-based alloys are to be used. All investments should be heat soaked for 30 minutes to ensure an even

temperature throughout the mould. When investment is heated the wax first softens, then melts, after which it boils before igniting. During these phases some wax is absorbed by the investment to form an impermeable carbon deposit on the surface of the mould. This layer prevents the mould gases escaping unless it is eliminated by an adequate heat soak.

Casting machines

There are two basic types of casting machine, those using steam to force metal into the mould and those using centrifugal force. These machines are operated mechanically or electrically, but only the mechanically operated machines will be described here.

Steam pressure casting. A typical steam casting machine is the Solbrig (Fig. 3.3).

1   The container is removed from the moveable arm, lined to a

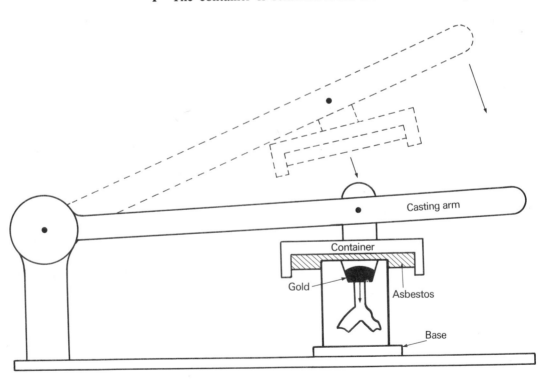

Fig. 3.3   A Solbrig casting machine.

depth of 5 mm with asbestos and left covered with water for 30 minutes. After this period the excess water is absorbed with a paper towel until moderate thumb pressure just causes moisture to ooze around the thumb. The lid is then attached to the casting arm and the correct-sized cylinder holder selected for the base.

2   The preheated casting cylinder is removed from the furnace and placed on the base of the casting machine. Gold alloy is placed in the crucible formed in the investment and the metal heated with a blow-torch flame until it begins to collapse, at which point a little flux is added (see Appendix). Flux should not be added before the metal collapses and covers the sprue hole, otherwise it might enter the hole and block it. Care should be taken to add only the minimum amount necessary to keep the surface of the metal clean. The metal is heated until it takes on a spherical shape and begins to rotate or spin. The asbestos is then brought down onto the hot casting cylinder and held firmly in position for 30 seconds, during which time steam forms and forces molten metal into the mould. If melting takes longer than 1 minute, the casting cylinder should be replaced in the furnace to heat soak for a further 10 minutes whilst the cause of the delay is determined. To cast before the metal is completely molten invariably results in an incomplete casting with rounded margins. Strict observance of the condition of the alloy when melting is of paramount importance.

3   When the casting arm is raised, the excess metal is seen as a flat button of metal on the inverted base of the crucible. This button is allowed to cool until the metal loses its red glow to become a dull metallic colour and the casting cylinder is then quenched in cold water.

Centrifugal casting.   For safety reasons, a horizontally mounted centrifugal casting machine must be firmly bolted inside a well (which can be made of brick and concrete or asbestos and wood), so that if any part of the machine or its contents should become dislodged during the casting procedure it will be contained within the well.

The centrifugal casting machine consists of two arms which meet at a central spindle. One arm contains a cradle for holding the casting cylinder and a crucible in which the metal is melted, whilst the other carries a moveable weight used to balance the machine (Fig. 3.4). It is powered by a spring in the base (see Appendix).

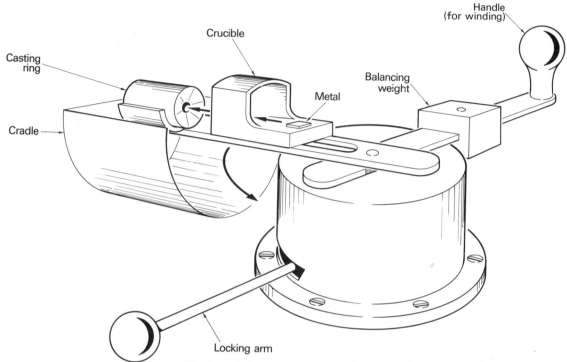

Fig. 3.4 A horizontally mounted centrifugal casting machine.

1 All components, casting cylinder, crucible and metal, are assembled onto the casting machine and the balancing weight adjusted, to ensure even spin.

2 The casting cylinder, crucible and metal are removed and heated in a furnace as described.

3 Meanwhile the spring is wound; the balancing arm being moved to the point at which the pressure of the spring can just be felt, and given three or four turns. The locking arm is lifted into the notch in the casting machine to lock the machine in position.

4 The blow torch is set (Fig. 3.5).

5 The preheated crucible, loaded with metal, is positioned in the casting machine with the open end facing the operator. A metal instrument is used to adjust the position of the metal to the top of the inclined floor of the crucible. The cylinder is placed in the cradle with the sprue hole towards the crucible as illustrated (Fig. 3.4). The crucible is slid along the casting arm until it lies firmly against the cylinder.

6 Heating of the metal with a blow torch is started immediately. As the metal begins to melt the edges curl and it starts to slide down the inclined floor of the crucible. Flux is added at this point. Eventually the metal assumes the shape of a sphere and begins to spin, at which stage the locking arm is withdrawn from the casting machine but held in the horizontal position. When the metal reaches complete fluidity the flame is removed and simultaneously the locking arm is released to spin the machine and the centrifugal force causes the metal to be flung into the mould.

Centrifugal castings are denser than those cast by steam pressure because centrifugal force produces a controlled pressure whilst steam depends upon the arbitrary moisture content of the asbestos.

Melting the metal

Metal (for types of alloy see Appendix) may be melted by gas (town or natural gas) with compressed air or oxygen, by electric arc, or induction coil.

Gas and compressed air

This is used almost exclusively for melting alloys with a melting range below 1000°C. Various torches are available and controls differ but in principle the procedure is as follows:

1 Gas and air tube connections are checked. The gas control on the torch is turned to the fully open position, the trigger depressed and the gas turned on and ignited. The flame length is adjusted so that when the trigger is released a small pilot flame remains.

2 The air control is left in the fully open position at all times, the pressure being adjusted at the bench tap. This prevents a build up of pressure inside the pipe line, during the casting procedure, which could fracture the pipe.

3 The flame is set as shown in Fig. 3.5, the reducing zone being

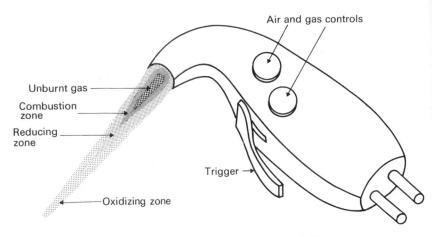

Air and gas controls

Unburnt gas

Combustion
zone

Reducing
zone

Trigger →

Oxidizing zone

Fig. 3.5 Blow torch for town
gas and compressed air.

used because the intense heat melts the metal quickly and prevents
oxidation of the alloy.

4   After loading the casting machine, the hand holding the torch is
positioned to the side of the crucible, not directly in front of it, to
prevent a throwback of heat onto the back of the operator's hand.
The flame is not played on one spot but is moved over the metal to
prevent overheating of isolated areas. A dull appearance of the metal
indicates incorrect use of the blow-torch flame causing the metal to
oxidize whereas correct heating, using the reducing zone, produces a
shiny appearance. As the metal spins it is cast into the mould, the air
is turned off at the bench, the trigger released on the blow torch and
the gas turned off at the casting bench.

Gas and oxygen

The gas–oxygen torch is used mainly for melting alloys of high
fusing temperatures, in the region of 1300°C. The torch consists of a
single jet nozzle and a single gas control, the oxygen being
controlled from the valve on the top of the oxygen bottle. Coloured
protective goggles should be worn by the operator and onlookers.

1   The gas and oxygen tubes are attached to their respective
connectors, the gas turned on and ignited and the oxygen adjusted to
70 000–105 000 N/m² (10–15 psi). The gas control knob on the
torch is adjusted to produce a light blue jet about 2·5 cm long with a
gentle hissing sound coming from the torch.

2 After loading the centrifugal casting machine (steam pressure is not used when casting the higher fusing alloys), the area just outside the light blue zone of the flame is brushed over the metal. As the alloy melts (usually in about 30 seconds) it becomes spherical and shiny. It is cast into the mould immediately it becomes molten.

3 The oxygen is turned off and allowed to clear the pipeline before the gas is turned off.

4 The alloy is bench cooled.

Electric arc melting apparatus

This apparatus generally consists of a control cabinet attached to a 30-amp power point and two-carbon electrodes with leads from the control cabinet. With the power switched on, the electrodes are brought into contact to produce around their ends a brilliant electric arc which is used to melt the higher fusing gold alloys and cobalt–chromium based alloys. This arc can damage eyes and skin if a protective mask is not worn, therefore the manufacturer's instructions should be followed closely. If there is any doubt about the correct technique to be used the manufacturer should be contacted before using the apparatus. The following technique is given as a general guide only and should not be used in preference to a manufacturer's instructions (see Appendix).

1 A current is selected according to the alloy being melted, as indicated by the manufacturer's instructions. One electrode is attached to the selected negative terminal on the control panel, the other to the positive terminal. The electrodes are set at approximately 10 cm in length, and about 5 cm apart.

2 A safety foot switch is incorporated in the circuit and an arc cannot be produced until this is activated, which must not be until safety procedures have been followed.

3 A specially designed safety visor is placed on the head and the centrifugal casting machine loaded.

4 A foot is placed ready to depress the safety switch and the protective visor pulled over the face. The operator is unable to see through the visor until the arc has been set. The trigger control is squeezed to bring the carbon electrodes into contact and the foot switch depressed. A brilliant arc is produced around the end of the electrodes, which are positioned about 3–4 mm apart when pressure on the trigger is slightly released.

5   The electrodes are held 12 mm away from the metal. High fusing gold alloys do not spin but the ingots become rounded and then join together to form a sphere. They are cast immediately the sphere is formed, which takes no longer than 30 seconds. Base metal alloys used in the porcelain bonded to metal technique are cast when the outer edges of the ingots become rounded, a slight dross always being left in the crucible.

6   After casting, the trigger is released to break the arc and the foot removed from the safety switch. The protective visor is then removed and the machine switched off.

The electric arc melting apparatus should be kept in a room which is locked during operation, preferably without windows or with them covered with an opaque film so that there is no danger of accidental observation of the arc by people not wearing a protective visor. There is no known danger to the operator as long as the safety precautions are followed.

Cleaning the casting

The casting should be left in the investment for 3–5 minutes until the button loses its redness, after which it is quenched by total immersion in cold water. Quenching produces castings of fine grain structure which exhibit annealed properties. The violent action of quenching causes the investment to disintegrate and facilitates the removal of the casting. A wax knife is run around the inside of the cylinder, keeping it well away from the casting, until the bulk of the investment and casting can be pushed out. The bulk of the investment is prised off the casting, care being taken to avoid damage to the margins, and the remainder brushed off under running water.

Removal of oxides

Most gold castings exhibit a dull oxidized surface. This is removed by 'pickling' the castings in a dilute solution of hydrochloric or sulphuric acid, the dilution used generally being 50% acid, 50% water. A dilute solution of nitric acid can be used for badly stained castings. Normal safety precautions should be taken with acids.

1 The casting is placed in a pyrex evaporating dish, covered with acid solution, and gently heated over a Bunsen burner flame. It should not be allowed to boil.

2 To prevent contamination of the acid or casting a pair of plastic-coated tweezers are used to remove the clean casting from the solution, and the casting rinsed under cold running water.

3 Very dark castings are generally indicative of an inadequate burnout time of the mould, the discoloration being removed by sulphuric acid. Stubborn discoloration may be removed by nitric acid.

A modern and safer method for removing oxides is by use of an ultrasonic cleaner. The casting is placed in a detergent solution in the ultrasonic bath, and ultrasonic vibrations act upon the surface of the metal to form bubbles. The vibratory waves remove the oxides and investment from the casting. Ten minutes in the ultrasonic bath is usually sufficient to clean a casting, a longer period being allowed for removal of stubborn stains.

Casting failures

Failure to obtain a perfect casting is generally caused by a deviation from the correct technique. Below are listed common faults together with their causes.

Surface nodules may be found anywhere on the casting and are due to faulty investing technique, which allows air bubbles to remain on the surface of the wax pattern. The air bubbles fill with metal and become nodules when the metal is cast.

Small ridges are caused by movement of the casting cylinder before the investment has set and may be found on any surface of the casting.

Fins or fine feathery ridges may also be found anywhere on the casting, and are caused by too rapid heating, which vaporizes the water in the investment too rapidly and cracks the surface of the mould.

Rough castings may be caused by:
1   Direct wax patterns inadequately cleansed of traces of blood and saliva
2   Overheating of the mould or metal causing the gypsum binder to decompose in the presence of carbon at temperatures above 700°C, the resultant disintegration causing the roughness
3   High casting pressures resulting in a damaged mould, generally caused by overwinding of the centrifugal casting machine.

Foreign body inclusions, usually investment or superfluous flux, are found in areas furthest from the point of sprue attachment.

Distorted casting. Distortion is generally found at the gingival margin or proximal boxes, especially with a M.O.D. casting, and may be caused by faulty impressions or casts, insufficient care when removing the pattern from the die, or failure to invest immediately the pattern has been removed. Failure to use a liner in the casting cylinder and insufficient heating of the mould can also be a source of distortion.

Porosity is the reduction in density of a casting by the presence of voids, due to the absorption of mould gases and the lack of precautions to compensate for alloy contraction.

   a   Localized porosity is found in the region of sprue attachment (Fig. 3.6) and is the result of thin sprues or sprueing to thin areas.
   b   Subsurface porosity (Fig. 3.6), caused by high mould temperature or overheated alloy, becomes apparent as the surface is polished during the finishing stage.
   c   Backpressure porosity is found at the extremities of the casting (Fig. 3.6) where gases are slow to vacate the mould and build up pressure at the extremities, preventing complete filling of the mould.

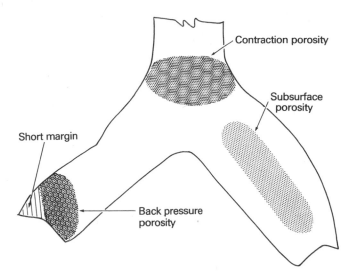

Fig. 3.6   Casting failures.

Incomplete castings are the result of gases in the mould causing backpressure, insufficiently heated, or incompletely melted metal. During prolonged melting the mould can cool sufficiently to cause the metal to solidify before complete filling.

FINISHING

When the casting has been cleaned of investment and oxides it is finished to a high lustre in the following manner.

1   The sprues and button are removed using a piercing saw, the cut being made close to the casting to reduce wastage of metal, and the area reshaped using a 22-mm carborundum cut-off disc.

2   Before the casting is tried on the die, the fitting surface is scrutinized for the presence of surface irregularities, those present being removed by a No. 3 round bur. The casting is then fitted onto the die and need not be removed until polishing has been completed.

3   Irregularities on the surface to be polished are removed by a No. 3 round bur. These irregularities should be minimal if investing has been carried out correctly. A pear-shaped finishing bur is used to develop the grooves. A new bur cuts quickly whereas a well-used one burnishes. Abrasive wheels, such as carborundum should not be

used unless recontouring is required because they scratch the surface, thus increasing the time required to obtain a smooth finish.

4   The casting is smoothed using a hard rubber wheel, such as Wipla W50. It must be moved over the metal continually, using a rotary movement to prevent formation of facets. A softer rubber wheel may be used to smooth the metal further if desired.

5   Polishing is carried out using felt wheels and an abrasive compound. (Although special felt polishing wheels can be purchased usually 2·5 cm in diameter, they can be made from a felt cone at a fraction of the cost.) On rotating the felt wheel the abrasive is incorporated and polishing continued in the manner described for the rubber wheel. To polish the grooves a bristle brush, impregnated with abrasive compound is jabbed sharply into them. A clean felt wheel and bristle brush are impregnated with jeweller's rouge and the polishing process repeated (see Appendix).

6   Finally, a clean wool polishing mop is rotated over the whole of the casting to give a high gloss. All polishing compound is removed with hot detergent or in an ultrasonic cleaner, after which the casting is rinsed under running water.

HEAT TREATMENTS

To minimize the marginal cement line and percolation, the margins of a cast restoration are burnished to the tooth; this requires a homogenized grain structure. Since the heat generated during polishing causes non-homogeneous grain structure this must be reversed by heating the alloy to obtain a reorientation of its grain structure. There are two types of heat treatment: annealing or homogenization which softens the alloy, and precipitation which hardens it (see Appendix).

Annealing

The following treatment is carried out after the finishing procedure has been completed. The casting is placed on a piece of asbestos, or a refractory tray kept for the purpose and placed in a preheated furnace at 700°C. This temperature is maintained for 3–4 minutes, by which time the metal should be cherry red in colour. A bowl of cold water is placed near the furnace door, the asbestos lifted out of the furnace and the casting dropped into the water. The annealed casting is pickled to remove the surface oxides.

Precipitation hardening

Alloys may be hardened in air or in a salt bath. The technique recommended by the manufacturer for a particular alloy should be followed closely, but when no instructions are given the following procedures may be helpful.

Hardening in air

The casting furnace is preheated to 450°C before placing the casting in the furnace on an asbestos or refractory tray. The furnace is allowed to cool to 250°C over a period of 30 minutes, when the casting is quenched.

If cooling is too slow the restoration may be devoid of ductility, yet if it cools too quickly the maximum strength will not be attained (see Appendix).

Salt baths

Salt baths produce better physical properties, prevent oxidation of the surface of the alloy, are inexpensive, effective and can be used repeatedly. Castings should be dry when placed into the bath because introduction of water produces violent explosion.

Equal parts of potassium nitrate and sodium nitrate salts are mixed and heated in a double pan, until they become liquid, at about 200°C. The temperature of the liquid is then raised to 400°C before placing the dry casting in the solution. At this point the pan is removed from the source of heat and the liquid allowed to cool to 250°C before the casting is removed.

4 Bridges

A dental bridge is an appliance constructed to replace one or more missing teeth, thus restoring masticatory efficiency and improving the patient's appearance. Usually a bridge is fixed in place so that the patient cannot remove it; this distinguishes it from a partial denture which is removeable.

Diagnosis and treatment planning by the dentist takes into account the condition and number of teeth. the condition of the periodontal tissues and state of the alveolar bone as determined by radiographic examination, the occlusion including partial dentures if present, the state of oral hygiene and the attitude of the patient to dentistry in general and bridge construction in particular. Any preliminary treatment considered necessary should be completed before work on a bridge is started.

Study casts

Upper and lower alginate impressions are taken for the construction of study casts (see Chapter 1). When correctly mounted on an articulator, study casts allow a thorough study of the occlusion from every angle, including the lingual aspect which is not visible in the mouth. Any cuspal locking and occlusal paths are noted. Study of edentulous areas helps to indicate the most suitable type of pontic. The angulation of the teeth may be studied on a parallelometer with reference to the feasibility of parallelism between abutment teeth. Various designs may be cut and waxed on a duplicate cast to determine the most suitable bridge, which may be shown to the patient for his approval and to enhance his appreciation of the lengthy and expensive laboratory procedures of which he may be unaware. At this stage the dentist may discuss the case with the technician, and may invite him to see the patient to provide a better understanding of, and personal interest in, the case than could be obtained from a set of casts.

If large and multiple edentulous areas are bridged, the increased stress on the abutment teeth may be harmful to the supporting tissues, so a partial denture is also considered. As a rule, an abutment tooth can support double the load normally carried. Postextraction resorption is often an important factor in deciding whether a bridge or a denture is indicated.

The factors which govern the choice of bridge include the clinical condition of the teeth being considered and the size of the pulp chambers. Where possible, teeth which necessarily require restoration are used in preference to sound ones. The length of the clinical crown greatly influences the retention available. The position of the abutments in the dental arch and their degree of parallelism, coupled with the size of the edentulous area, all determine the choice of abutment teeth and the design of the bridge.

Retainer selection

Retainers generally used in bridge construction are the M.O.D. with capped cusps, the three-quarter crown or partial veneer crown, the full veneer crown, intra-radicular posts, and modified class III and IV inlays. This subject is dealt with in clinical texts.

Pontic selection

Ideally pontics should be harmless to the oral tissues, aesthetically acceptable and easily cleaned, as well as restoring masticatory efficiency. With the exception of the all-porcelain bridge, pontics are constructed in metal or metal faced with either porcelain or acrylic resin. The all-metal pontic is used posteriorly, facings being added when appearance is important.

Pontic selection therefore involves decisions on whether a facing should be used and which type should be chosen, and consideration of its effect upon the metal design. Some commercially available facings are the Steele's flat-back facing, the Steele's

Trupontic facing, the long-pin facing and the stock porcelain denture tooth. Facings constructed in the laboratory are: porcelain bonded to metal, acrylic retained on metal and the 20° angle facing.

Factors governing selection of facing are the availability, cost, the amount of alveolar bone resorption, the importance of appearance, the length of the edentulous span and the occlusal forces present. Most commercially produced facings require protection of the incisal edge or occlusal surface, and metal is used which increases the strength of the bridge but detracts from its appearance. Fortunately it is possible to make individual pontics (custom built) using porcelain bonded to metal, combining aesthetics with strength.

Bridge design

A bridge comprises the following components (Fig. 4.1):

Abutment   A tooth specially prepared to support and retain the bridge.

Pier   An intermediate abutment tooth used as a centre support in a long span bridge.

Retainer   A restoration constructed to fit the prepared abutment tooth.

Pontic   The part of the bridge which replaces a lost natural tooth.

Connector   This joins the component parts of the bridge.

The design of a bridge is considered in conjunction with the choice of abutments; the various designs are as follows:

The fixed–fixed bridge.   This is supported by retainers on each side

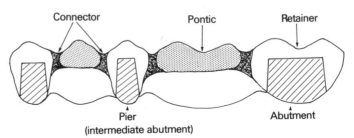

Fig. 4.1   Component parts of a bridge.

of the edentulous area. The retainers must have the same line of insertion (Fig. 4.2A).

The fixed–movable bridge is also supported by retainers on each side of the edentulous area, but one retainer is modified by the incorporation of an attachment which allows a limited amount of movement within the retainer (Fig. 4.2B). This method permits the retainers to have different lines of insertion.

The cantilever bridge. The pontic is supported on only one side (Fig. 4.2C).

The spring–cantilever bridge. Other teeth intervene between the pontic and its retainers to which the pontic is attached by a palatal or lingual bar (Fig. 4.2D).

Study bridge

When the design of the bridge has been decided, a mock-up known as a 'study bridge' may be made on a duplicate study cast. The preparations are cut to determine parallelism and position of proximal margins, the bridge is waxed using an acrylic resin tooth as the pontic. This may be shown to the patient to explain what is to be done.

Temporary bridge

Before preparation of the abutment teeth, consideration is given to temporary coverage of them and maintenance of the various

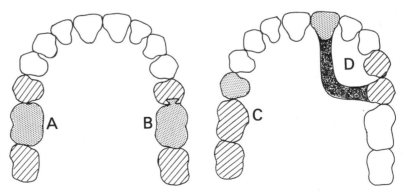

Fig. 4.2 Bridge designs: (A) fixed–fixed; (B) fixed–movable; (C) cantilever; (D) spring cantilever.

interdental relationships. This is accomplished by the construction of a temporary bridge, a convenient time to take the impression for this being in the period whilst awaiting anaesthesia.

An acrylic denture tooth is trimmed to fit the edentulous area and positioned in the mouth by the aid of pieces of carding wax. An alginate impression in a stock tray is taken and placed in a selfseal polythene bag. The plastic tooth usually comes away in the impression, but if not it is removed from the mouth. The abutment teeth are prepared and the appropriate impressions and occlusal registrations taken. The alginate impression is taken from the polythene bag, dried, and the pontic area and the impression of the abutment teeth filled with a suitable temporary bridge material such as Sevriton (see Appendix). The surrounding tissues are lightly lubricated with petroleum jelly and the impression reinserted and correctly seated in the mouth. It is left until the resin becomes warm, when it is removed before the heat damages the tissues. After polymerization is complete the margins are trimmed and polished, and the bridge is set in place with zinc oxide–eugenol cement.

Impressions and working casts

The choice of a rubber-base impression material eliminates the necessity to localize dies, thus ensuring accurate working casts. An impression of the palate is not required unless a spring–cantilever bridge is to be constructed.

Casts are poured in die stone and based with an equal mix of plaster of Paris and Kaffir 'D' (see Chapter 1). After removal of the impression from the cast it is cleansed of casting debris and left to stand for 15 minutes to allow the elastic memory to readjust the material. A second cast is then prepared; this is used to localize the component parts of the bridge prior to soldering. Theoretically, dowel pins are not required in the second cast but, in case of accidental damage to the first cast, it is useful to incorporate them.

Prescription

There is a growing tendency for the dental surgeon to send his

PRESCRIPTION

| Dental surgeon's name and address | | Laboratory No: |
| Patient's name | | National Health No: |

Place a tick in the appropriate box below

| Special tray | | Study cast | | |

Inlay	Direct		Crown	A.J.C.		Cast core		Laboratory use only
	Indirect			P.J.C.		Bridge		
				Gold		Splint		

Tooth	Preparation	Tooth	Preparation

BRIDGES

Design and comments:

Date required:

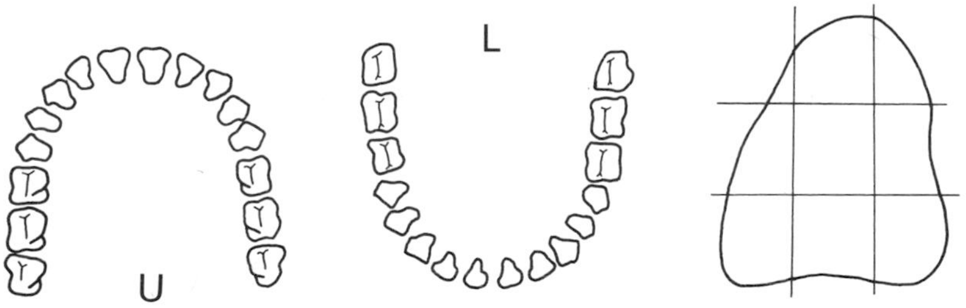

Fig. 4.3 A typical prescription chart required when work is sent to a laboratory

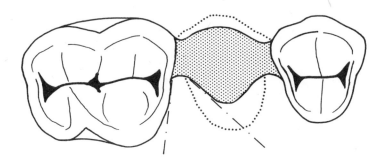

Fig. 4.4 The buccolingual width of a pontic is narrowed to reduce the occlusal forces transmitted to the abutment teeth. The greatest reduction should be on the lingual aspect. The embrasures are also widened.

technical work to a commercial laboratory instead of employing a technician in his practice. It is therefore all the more important that a comprehensive prescription is sent to the laboratory, to ensure that the appliance is constructed to his precise requirements. A typical prescription chart appears in (Fig. 4.3).

PONTIC CONSTRUCTION

The general principles to be considered and followed in pontic

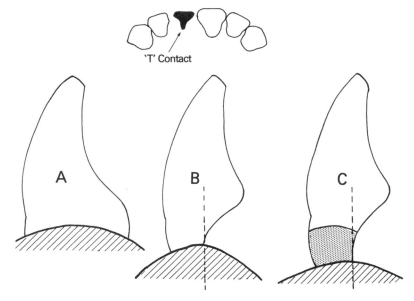

'T' Contact

Fig. 4.5 The labiolingual width of the pontic is narrowed.
(A) Gingival contour in the natural dentition. (B) Normal contour after resorption.
(C) Excessive gingival resorption. Shaded area is stained to simulate cementation or gingival tissue. When ridge lapping, the facing must contact the tissue up to the centre of the ridge to form a 'T' contact, after which it should develop a large easily cleaned area.

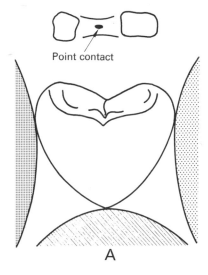

Point contact

A

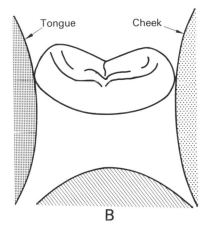

Tongue   Cheek

B

Fig. 4.6 (A) A posterior pontic should contact the tissue in one spot in the centre of the ridge known as a 'point' contact. (B) The all-metal pontic should have sufficient space beneath it to allow the tongue and cheek to clean the undersurface of the pontic.

construction are given below.

The faciolingual width of the pontic should be narrower than the same dimension of its natural predecessor to allow for the resorption of the alveolar process and to permit easier food shedding, thus reducing the occlusal load on the abutment teeth (Fig. 4.4).

The mesiodistal diameter of the facing should be slightly narrower than the same dimension of the edentulous area to allow for the positioning and shaping of the connector.

The height should harmonize with the dentition. Some difficulty may be experienced in the gingival area when considerable resorption has taken place, in which case the elongated neck of the facing may be stained to simulate cementum of the gingiva (Fig. 4.5).

The interstitial spaces, for reasons of hygiene, should be conical and wider than in the natural dentition (Fig. 4.4). Unfortunately, this is not always possible to achieve in the anterior region because of aesthetic requirements.

Protection of the incisal edge of commercial facings by capping with metal is necessary. Although these are generally referred to as *interchangeable facings* they are difficult to replace once damaged.

When ridge lapping, the mesiodistal contact with the alveolar ridge should be convex whilst buccolingually it should be spheroidal. The contact is therefore approximately T-shaped, and is called a 'T' contact. It covers the minimum of tissue at the same time as giving a good appearance (Fig. 4.5).

Posterior pontics should contact the tissue in one spot in the centre of the ridge, known as a 'point contact'. This is the most easily cleaned of the pontic designs (Fig. 4.6A).

The all-metal pontic, often incorrectly referred to as the sanitary or selfcleansing pontic, should be constructed with sufficient space above the tissue to allow the tongue and cheeks to keep the undersurface of the pontic clean or, at least, to allow adequate access for a toothbrush or interdental stimulator (Fig. 4.6B).

The method of constructing the most commonly used pontics is described in the following pages.

All-gold pontic

An all-gold pontic is generally confined to the posterior region of the mouth, where appearance is not a consideration. Since an easily cleaned area must exist below the pontic, this type cannot be used when the clinical crowns of the abutment teeth are short.

1   An acrylic resin denture tooth may be used to form the pontic, but these are too costly for this purpose and take longer than wax to burn out of the investment mould. An efficient method is to pour inlay wax into various sized silicone moulds (see Appendix) to obtain a stock with a wide selection of pontics. A wax pontic of compatible mesiodistal width is selected to fit between the waxed retainers and the cuspal angles reduced to prevent cuspal locking and to facilitate food shedding, thereby reducing the occlusal load on the abutment teeth. Wax from the gingival area is removed until the pontic is about 3 mm thick, and oval when viewed from a proximal surface. There should be no sharp angles on which the tongue or cheeks may rub. The undersurface of the pattern, when viewed from the lingual or buccal aspect, should be approximately parallel to the occlusal surface, to give the pontic an oval cylindrical shape.

2   To support the pattern whilst adjusting the occlusal contour to the opposing cast, a piece of carding wax or plasticine is adapted to the edentulous area and lubricated before positioning the pattern.

3   Whilst adjusting the occlusal surface the spillways are defined to allow food to spill (shed) from the occlusal surface immediately pressure builds up, thereby reducing the stress applied to the abutment teeth. By narrowing the buccolingual dimension of the pontic, a further reduction of the occlusal load upon the abutment teeth is possible.

4   The embrasures should be widened to facilitate cleaning and to assist with food deflection which, if correctly directed, can be a source of stimulation to the periodontal tissues, ensuring an adequate blood supply to the edentulous area to maintain healthy soft tissue and bone (Fig. 4.4). The bulk of the reduction should be made on the lingual aspect, since a reduction of more than 1 mm on the buccal aspect can cause the patient to bite his cheek (Fig. 4.4).

Molars should be reduced to the buccolingual width of a premolar, whereas premolars should be reduced by about one-third.

5   It should be remembered that this pattern is thick and will require a sprue former of at least 3 mm diameter. It is important that the pontic is porosity free to avoid adhesion of plaque.

Gold with a commercial facing

The Steele's trupontic may be used in the anterior and posterior regions of the mouth, but its bulk restricts its use to areas where considerable alveolar resorption has taken place. A posterior trupontic will be described.

1   A facing is selected which is slightly narrower than the mesiodistal width of the edentulous area to allow for the connectors, and slightly longer occlusogingivally than the adjacent teeth to allow for contouring.

2   The gingival area is ground to produce a point contact with the tissue. When appearance is important the pontic is ridge lapped. After grinding, the occlusal surface must be 3 mm below the occlusal table of the natural dentition to allow space for a gold occlusal surface. The buccolingual aspect is reduced if necessary and further reduction may be needed to widen the embrasures.

3   After modification, the angles around the occlusal surface are chamfered to allow for metal protection (Fig. 4.7) and the facing waxed in position on the master cast. The waxed retainers are removed from the dies and the buccal aspect of the cast lubricated with petroleum jelly. A thick mix of plaster is formed into a block over the buccal aspect of the adjacent teeth and facing, care being taken to avoid damage to the margins of the abutment teeth (Fig. 4.8). When the plaster has set it is removed, trimmed and the master cast and facing cleaned.

4   After lubricating the facing, inlay wax is poured into the retentive groove and pressure exerted as it solidifies. The excess is removed and a pointed instrument used to ease the wax carefully out of the groove. The facing is relubricated, the wax rod inserted into the groove and a piece of sheet casting wax adapted to the occlusal surface. The two waxes are sealed together by the use of a warm Le

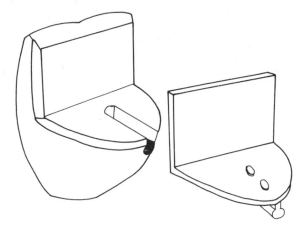

Fig. 4.7 Steele's trupontic. The outer edge of the metal bearing area must be chamfered. A metal backing may be used.

Cron carver. Peripheral excess is removed and the occlusal surface built in wax.

(An alternative method is to incorporate a prefabricated metal backing to the facing (Fig. 4.7). When the facing has been contoured a metal backing is selected and trimmed to the edge of the facing with scissors. Using an alumina stone it is more accurately trimmed to the inner edge of the chamfer cut around the facing. The outer end of the retentive pin is reduced by 0·5 mm to allow for a peripheral layer of gold. Inlay wax is added to the protrusions on the surface of the metal backing and pressure exerted as it solidifies. The occlusal surface is then waxed.)

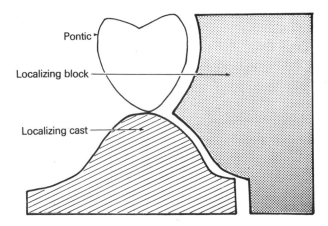

Fig. 4.8 Plaster localizing block. Care must be taken not to damage the margins of the dies.

5 After sprueing, the facing is withdrawn from the pattern. A piece of sticky wax is softened and held against the buccal surface of the facing until it solidifies. Holding the sticky wax in one hand and the sprue and pattern in the other, they are carefully drawn apart.

6 The pattern is invested and cast in the usual way. The casting is finished to the rubber wheel stage, the facing checked for fit and, after completion of minor adjustments to ensure accurate fit and shape, the metal is polished.

7 The glaze remaining after contouring is removed from the facing which is then washed thoroughly, and the whole facing reglazed so that glazing is even over the whole area. Since commercial facings fuse around 1400°C it is difficult to reglaze in modern laboratory porcelain furnaces, so a special glazing medium has to be used (see Appendix). To facilitate manipulation, a pair of tweezers is modified by soldering a Steele's metal backing to them. The facing is then held by its retentive groove on the metal backing. An even layer of glazing medium, mixed to a creamy consistency is painted onto the unglazed surfaces and the facing gently vibrated. If carefully heated over a Bunsen burner flame the medium will turn white, thus revealing any uncovered areas, which are then coated. The facing is heated in the doorway of a preheated furnace at 900°C for 5 minutes before being placed in the furnace and fired for 2 to 3 minutes. It is cooled in air. If correctly glazed the surface will be smooth; pits indicate an uneven application of glaze, and a milky appearance the application of too thick a layer. In either case the glaze should be removed and the process repeated correctly.

The Steele's flat-back facing is inserted onto the pontic from an incisal direction which precludes the possibility of the incisal edge being capped with metal, thereby limiting its use to cases where stress will not be too great, for example where there is a large overjet or an opposing denture. Being thin, this facing is used where the adjacent anterior crowns are thin labiolingually.

1 The edentulous area of the cast is blackened with carbon from a pencil lead, which will transfer to the contacting areas of the facing when it is positioned on the cast, thus indicating where the porcelain is to be removed to allow accurate fitting to ridge lap the cast. The labial surface is reshaped as required.

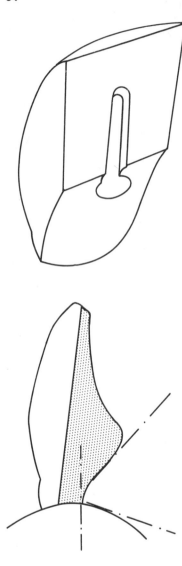

Fig. 4.9 Steele's flat back. The porcelain and metal backing form a 'T' contact with the tissue. The cingulum is kept away from the tissue to form a wide easily cleansed area.

2 After adjustment the facing is waxed in position and a plaster overbite formed.

3 The lingual and proximal angles are chamfered, but not the incisal, and a metal backing ground to fit 1 mm within the confines of the facing.

4 The master cast is lubricated and the lingual aspect of the pontic built in wax. Care should be taken during the waxing procedure to prevent inlay wax running onto the adjacent previously-carved retainers and spoiling them. If considered necessary this may be avoided by laying a piece of lubricated tissue paper against the surface of the retainers. The wax and facing should form a 'T' contact with the tissue, the facing being the cross member, whilst the wax, being the vertical member, maintains contact with the tissue to the crest of the ridge (Fig. 4.9). The lingual interstitial spaces are widened and the cingulum kept away from the tissue to form a wide, easily-cleaned space. Reduction of the lingual aspect allows stimulation of the tissues and reduces the occlusal forces.

5 An important area requiring special attention is the junction between facing and wax in the gingival area. It is one of the hardest places to keep clean once the bridge has been fitted in the mouth, so the wax pattern should be a perfect fit against the facing and be very smooth.

6 A sprue former is attached to the cingulum and the facing removed and re-glazed whilst the pattern is cast.

The long-pin facing contains two long parallel pins which have a labiolingual path of insertion (Fig. 4.10). Its use is confined to the posterior region of the mouth or to anterior dentitions with wide labiolingual dimensions. The retentive pins should not be shortened, but the facing may be modified into a trupontic shape by the addition of porcelain.

1 The facing is contoured to give a 'T' contact on the master cast and a plaster overbite constructed.

2 Parallelism of the pins is important and the ends must be smooth. After lubrication of the facing, sheet casting wax is adapted to it with the pins protruding through the wax. The lingual surface is then built in inlay wax. When contouring the lingual surface the cingulum is trimmed with the ends of the pins just visible to assist

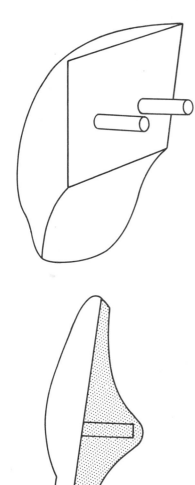

Fig. 4.10   Long-pin facing.

with accurate positioning of stainless steel pins at a later stage.

3   The pattern is sprued at the cingulum with the ends of the pins still visible, and the facing withdrawn from the pattern. It is important that the pin holes in the pattern are accurately reproduced in the metal, and this is ensured by inserting carbon rods or stainless steel wire, of the same diameter as the metal pins, into the holes in the pattern. Steel wire is preferable because when heated it carbonizes, acting as an antiflux preventing gold bonding to it, so that when removed from the casting an accurate hole results. Two straight 10-mm lengths of hard stainless steel wire are cut and the ends flattened and smoothed. These are inserted into the pattern until the ends are visible on the lingual aspect of the pattern indicating that the wire is at the end of the hole. The cingulum is thickened with wax in the area of the wire, final contouring being left until the pattern has been cast. A small ball of wax is also added to the extended ends of the wire to prevent it moving during investing.

4   After casting, but before removal of the sprues, the wires are removed one at a time. The wire is held with a pair of snipe-nosed pliers (and the button and sprues in the fingers) and slowly rotated to and fro until it is free to turn through 180° angle, when it is extracted from the casting.

5   The casting and facing are finished in the manner described for other facings.

A modified technique is the addition of porcelain to the gingival area of the long-pin facing to convert it into a long-pin trupontic (Fig. 4.11). Because of the difference in firing temperatures between the manufactured facing and the porcelains used in the laboratory, the chemical bond alone is not adequate, and undercuts are formed in the facing to give added retention.

1   Using a diamond wheel small undercuts are made on the lingual aspect of the facing in the gingival region.

2   The facing is placed on a pair of 'K' pliers (see Appendix) with the pins uppermost and behind the metal plate, the gingival area facing the tip of the pliers. Allowance is made for metal between the pins and the new porcelain. Vegetable oil is used to lubricate the pliers which are locked onto the facing.

3   After moistening the facing with water, the correct shade of

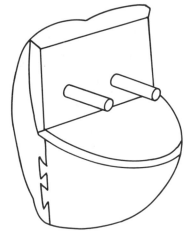

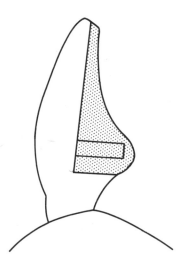

Fig. 4.11 Long-pin facing modified to a trupontic form. Retention is ground into the gingival area of the facing and porcelain fired onto this area.

porcelain is applied in the manner described for porcelain crowns (Chapter 5). It is built against the flat surface of the pliers and given a rounded gingival contour. The lock on the pliers is released, the facing carefully withdrawn from the pliers with a lateral sliding movement, and placed on a bed of silex crystals on a firing tray. Drying of the porcelain takes about 10 minutes in the doorway of the furnace before firing as described for porcelain jacket crowns.

4 The fused facing is trimmed to a spot or 'T' contact with the tissue as required, additions made where necessary, and then refired. When the contour fulfils as nearly as possible the general principles of pontic construction, the facing is coated with a glazing medium and refired. Finally the line angles round the facing are chamfered and the pontic constructed in the manner described.

A stock porcelain denture tooth may be used and has the advantages of being cheaper and more readily available than manufactured facings. This type of facing has a labiolingual path of insertion and the pins are considerably shorter than the long-pin facing, allowing it to be used in almost any pontic application.

1 A facing is selected and ground to harmonize with the natural dentition, and a plaster overbite constructed.

2 After chamfering of the lingual angles the pins are boxed with plaster, until the pins are barely covered. When set the plaster is trimmed using a scalpel, until the pins become faintly visible under the surface of the plaster.

3 The facing is lubricated, the lingual surface contoured in wax and the pattern cast and finished.

4 To improve retention the box in the casting is modified (Fig. 4.12). The proximal walls of the box are undercut by the use of an inverted cone bur. The plaster encasing the pins on the facing is removed and the pins bent slightly in a proximal direction. When the facing is cemented into the box extra retention will be obtained by the heads of the pins which spring slightly and engage in the undercuts in the box (Fig. 4.12).

Bonded porcelain pontics are increasingly popular because each pontic is made to the patient's individual shade and characteristics, the resultant appearance often being superior to that of manufactured facings. Good appearance is combined with strength,

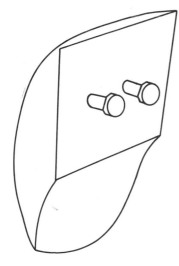

there is no cement line between facing and metal, and connectors may be covered with porcelain. These pontics may be soldered to conventional gold alloys. Gold is increasingly expensive but present developments in base metal alloys suggest that these may be used instead of gold thus reducing the cost. The bonded porcelain technique is described in Chapter 6.

The 20°-angle facing is possibly the most aesthetically pleasing of all porcelain facings, there being no gold visible on the labial or buccal aspects. Its name is taken from the angle of insertion of the facing in relation to the occlusal table (Fig. 4.13). It is most successfully used when the opposing dentition is a denture and when the clinical crowns of the abutment teeth are long.

1 An alumina tube of required diameter is selected and a piece

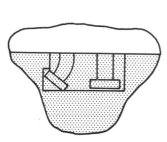

Fig. 4.12 (above) Porcelain denture tooth. The proximal walls of the box are undercut and the pins bent slightly in a proximal direction.

Fig. 4.13 (right) Construction of the porcelain section of a 20°-angle pontic. Its name is taken from the angle of insertion of the facing in relation to the occlusal table. (1) First layer of core material. (2) Second layer of core material.

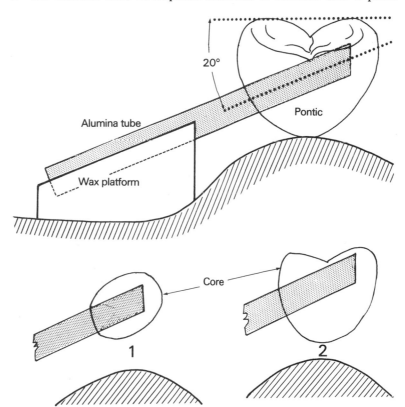

20–30 mm long is cut and ground to a slight angle at one end. The ground end of the tube is sealed with modelling wax and porcelain core material is built around it and about 4 mm along its length. This is placed on silex crystals and dried in the doorway of the furnace until all discoloration caused by the wax disappears. It is then fired in the normal way.

2   Modelling wax is softened and a platform is made in the palate of the master cast. The alumina tube is seated in the wax, at an angle of 20° to the occlusal table, with the cored end of the tube in the edentulous area, about 1 mm from the cast and 1 mm palatally off the line of the buccal walls of the abutments.

3   After removal of the tube, tissue paper is moistened and adapted to the pontic area; then the tube is reseated on the platform. Additional core material is added until the pontic is about 1 mm smaller than the required finished shape. The tube is then removed from the cast and the tissue paper peeled off the base of the facing, which is fired as before.

4   The core is ground to shape and covered with dentine and enamel porcelain which is fired, but not glazed. The shape is modified to accept a gold component, from which the pontic receives support and to which the retainers are soldered. Firstly the excess alumina tube is removed flush with the palatal surface of the facing. Then on one proximal surface 1 mm below the marginal ridge, a furrow 3 mm wide and 1·5–2·00 mm deep is cut around the palatal surface to the next proximal surface, the sides being given a slight taper (Fig. 4.14). The furrow is widened around the tube area until it finishes 1 mm above the gingival tissue. This gives the pontic added support. The periphery of the alumina tube is countersunk.

5   The modified facing is glazed.

6   The facing is lubricated and a preformed wax rod (see Chapter 2, intraradicular post) inserted into the alumina tube, the excess being cut away to leave 2 mm outside the facing. Inlay wax is used to recontour the proximal and lingual surfaces which are sealed to the wax rod. The rod is called the spigot and the proximal extensions are known as spurs. A metal sprue former is inserted into the wax spigot to strengthen it during the investing procedure and the pattern carefully withdrawn and invested. After casting in gold it is finished in the usual way.

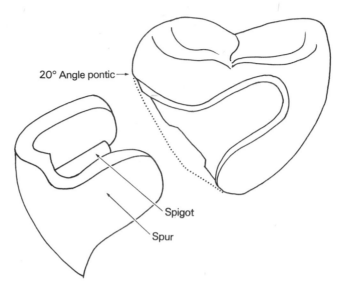

20° Angle pontic→

Spigot

Spur

Fig. 4.14 A 20°-angle pontic showing the porcelain prepared to accept the metal component.

7 When cementing the facing to the bridge, cement is placed on the spigot only and not down the alumina tube, otherwise pressure built in the tube will prevent the facing seating correctly on the spigot.

A twin-tube 20°-angle pontic can be used to overcome lack of parallelism between abutments. This is similar to the 20°-angle pontic, but two tubes are incorporated instead of one. The abutment teeth are prepared independently and a single spur and spigot attached to each retainer combine the units to form a bridge by use of the twin-tube pontic. Because of its bulk this facing is best suited to the molar region.

1 Two 3-cm lengths of alumina tube are bound together with a piece of platinum foil, the ends covered firstly with wax, then with core material, and fired in the manner described in the chapter on porcelain jacket crowns.

2 The pontic is constructed in the manner described for the single tube, and the proximal surfaces prepared to accept the spurs.

3 The spurs are made in two halves. Preformed wax rod is inserted into one tube and its corresponding spur formed in inlay wax. The spur is taken to the edge of the second tube and a ledge approximately 1 mm wide and 0·75 mm deep cut into it. At a later stage the second spur will sit on this ledge (Fig. 4.15).

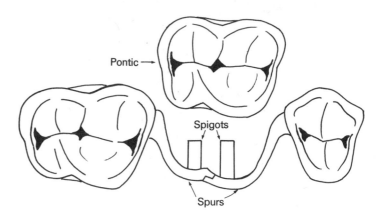

Fig. 4.15 Twin-tube 20°-angle pontic. The spurs are soldered to the retainers, the facing combining the units to form a bridge. The spurs meet and overlap between the two alumina tubes.

4   The pattern is invested, cast in gold and finished.

5   The spur is seated in the facing and lubricated. The second spur is then waxed to sit on the ledge in the first spur. This is sprued, cast and finished.

6   The finished spurs are soldered to their respective retainers and after cementation of the retainers the pontic is cemented to the bridge.

Acrylic resin.   The use of acrylic resin as a facing material declined for a number of years, mainly because of poor tissue response, too rapid wear and colour instability. New resins are becoming available which, according to their manufacturers, do not cause irritation of the tissues but, until this is proved clinically, it is advisable to form all tissue contact areas in highly polished metal.

1   The metal portion is constructed in the manner described for bonded porcelain pontics (Chapter 6), with the difference that the interface is reduced by a further 0·5 mm to allow room for retention pearls, and is extended gingivally to make contact with the tissue.

2   When the shape is considered suitable, the interface is coated with an adhesive and retention pearls sprinkled onto it (Fig. 4.16). These pearls eventually burn out with the wax pattern which is sprued, invested and cast as described. Since only the lower half of the pearls, now formed in metal and an integral part of the casting, are retentive, the top is ground off to make more space for the acrylic resin.

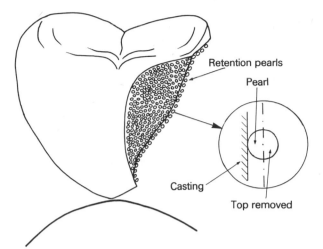

Retention pearls

Pearl

Casting

Top removed

Fig. 4.16 Acrylic resin as a facing. Plastic retention 'pearls' are sprinkled over the interface and burn out with the wax. after casting the top of the pearls are ground leaving the retentive lower half.

3 The interface is then masked by coating with an opacifier which is allowed to dry before the facing is contoured in non-residual wax.

4 The bridge is invested in plaster of Paris in a crown flask, packed with acrylic resin and polymerized (see Chapter 7).

5 Care should be exercised to prevent damage to the gold alloy when deflasking.

CONNECTORS

The pontic is attached to the retainer by means of a connector which may be solid, moveable or an extended bar. The rigid connector is oval in shape, similar to the contact area of the natural teeth to which it is analogous. It then deflects food without allowing stagnation areas around the gingiva, and can easily be cleaned. If it is necessary to contact the alveolar tissue, coverage should be minimal. To prevent tarnish and corrosion the alloys used for the connector should be similar to those used in the retainers.

Solid connectors

A solid connector may be cast, soldered or made of alumina (see porcelain bridge, page 98). When cast, it is an integral part of the bridge, being formed in wax, and the entire bridge cast in one piece. The soldered connector is formed in wax and cast as part of the pontic, after which it is soldered to the retainer. Both connectors should be kept well away from the gingiva, the normal contact area being the ideal position.

Cast connector

1 The waxed units are assembled on the localizing cast using the plaster overbite to position the pontic.
2 Inlay wax is used to seal the pontic to the retainer in the contact area, developing a wide embrasure and smooth oval shape.
3 After sprueing, the bridge is removed from the cast and the undersurface of the connector smoothly contoured with carding wax. The various connector positions and shapes are illustrated (Fig. 4.17).
4 The facing is removed and the bridge invested, cast and finished.

Soldered connectors

1 The units are assembled as described for the cast connector.
2 A piece of tissue paper lubricated with Teepol is adapted to the proximal surface of the retainer and the connector formed against it but attached to and continuous with the pontic. This forms a snug fit against the retainer whilst preventing adhesion.
3 The units are invested and cast separately, after which they are reassembled on the localizing cast in readiness for the soldering technique (see page 79).

Moveable connectors

There are two broad groups of moveable connector. One is the kind made in the laboratory to a dovetail design, and this will be described here. The other is manufactured commercially and connectors in this group are often referred to as precision attachments. This may be a misnomer because all dental laboratory productions are precisely constructed, so connectors in this second

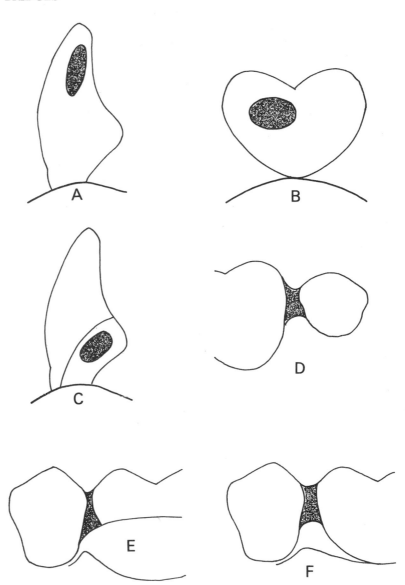

Fig. 4.17 Solid connectors should be oval in shape and be positioned in the area of the contact (A and B). If this is not possible it should be kept as far away from the gingiva as the bridge design will permit (C). They should form wide embrasures (D) and a smooth curvature with the undersurface of an all-gold pontic (E) or a rounded contour when the pontic contacts the tissue (F).

group are more accurately described as manufactured attachments. There are now many varieties and the subject has become so complex that it is too large to be discussed in a book of this size. The techniques involved require the highest standard of workmanship and only those fully conversant and practised in the techniques described in this book should contemplate undertaking such work.

Dovetail connector

This consists of two components, matrix and patrix. The patrix is the protrusive component attached to the pontic, whilst the matrix is the receptive part lying within the retainer (Fig. 4.18). A dovetail connector should be long in an incisogingival direction for retentive purposes, the walls of the matrix having a slight taper and being sufficiently thick to prevent distortion. The patrix should fit accurately into the matrix, and the isthmus joining the patrix to the pontic must be sufficiently large to impart rigidity.

1   The dental surgeon prepares the abutment tooth with a box adjacent to the endentulous area large enough to accommodate the attachment.

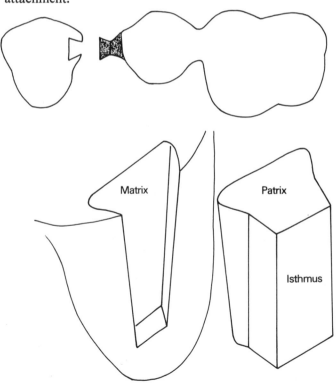

Fig. 4.18   The dovetail connector.

2 The retainer is waxed in the normal manner and the matrix formed by arbitrarily cutting the shape in the wax or by waxing around a mandril or carbon rod. Alternatively, the restoration may be cast to the normal shape and the shape of the matrix milled into it. Waxing around a mandril or carbon rod is the easiest and most accurate method. A number of mandrils can be prepared to varying widths and thicknesses which, when polished, produce smooth patterns (see Appendix).

3 The master cast is assembled on a parallelometer with the required mandril set at the same path of insertion as that of the other abutment. Sheet casting wax is adapted to the retainer and the lubricated mandril positioned within the pattern. Inlay wax is dripped around the mandril and the retainer contoured. The mandril is carefully withdrawn from the pattern which is sprued, invested and cast.

4 It is essential that the inside of the matrix is given a high polish during finishing. To accomplish this the bur end of a tapered fissure, bur, No. $\frac{1}{2}$, is encased in cotton wool, which is impregnated with polishing compound. The process is repeated with cotton wool impregnated with jewellers' rouge. The casting is thoroughly cleaned in an ultrasonic cleaner to remove every trace of polishing compound from the matrix.

5 The matrix is lubricated with Teepol and inlay wax adapted to it. A probe is warmed, inserted into the pattern and, with a gentle to-and-fro movement, the pattern is eased out of the matrix and examined for reproduction of detail. The pattern is replaced in the matrix and the probe removed by careful heating of the shank about 1 cm from the pattern.

6 All the bridge units are assembled on the localizing cast as described above. The proximal surface of the cast retainer is lubricated and the patrix sealed to the pontic by forming the isthmus. After sprueing, the patterns are carefully removed from the cast, invested, cast and finished.

Bar connectors

A bar connector, the spring cantilever arm, is used when the pontic is remote from the retainers. It must be rigid and, if very long, supported by rests on both sides of the pontic. Bar connectors should only minimally cover the gingival margins and not exert pressure upon them. They should be oval in shape and seated in the tissue, the depth depending upon the compressibility of the tissue. The fitting surface should be highly polished.

1   The retainers are cast and assembled on the localizing cast.

2   The gingival crevice of the posterior retainer is filled with wax, and then relieved by adapting a piece of No. 40 tin foil for a length of 3 mm along the bar. An outline of the bar, which should be 4 mm wide, is drawn on the cast and, in compliance with the dentist's instructions, the cast is scored. Starting 3 mm from the gingival margin of the retainer, plaster is removed to form a groove normally progressing to a depth of 0·5 mm at the bend in the arm and 2 mm at the edentulous area (Fig. 4.19).

3   The cast is lubricated and a piece of 0·4 mm sheet-casting wax, 3 mm wider than the bar, adapted to it and sealed along its periphery. This will prevent the wax lifting whilst the bar is built in inlay wax. Wax is added to a centre thickness of 3 mm and attached to the pontic so that the bar and pontic become indistinguishable. It

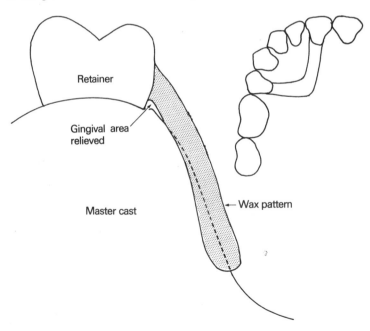

Fig. 4.19 The spring cantilever arm, showing how the arm is seated progressively deeper into the cast.

is contoured to blend with the retainer halfway up its lingual surface (Fig. 4.19). The excess peripheral wax is removed and the edges smoothed.

4 Long palatal bars have a tendency to warp so, after forming, the cast is lightly lubricated with petroleum jelly, the bar sprued (a large metal sprue at the bend in the arm and two auxiliary sprues, one at each end) and correctly seated on the cast. A mix of investment is painted over the bar and allowed to set. The partly-invested pattern is removed from the cast, assembled on a crucible former and further invested in the normal way.

5 When cast, the undersurface of the bar is given a high polish and the bridge assembled on the localizing cast in readiness for soldering.

PRINCIPLES OF SOLDERING

1 The castings to be soldered should be clean because solder will not flow over a dirty surface. After polishing, the units are pickled in hydrochloric acid or in an ultrasonic bath to free the surface of grease, and the soldering area sandpapered.

2 Units to be joined should be close, yet not touching. A very slight gap allows capillary attraction to draw the solder along the join.

3 The minimum of investment is used. Large investment blocks take a long time to heat, increasing the likelihood of oxidation of both solder and bridge, which prevents flow of the solder.

4 The join should be fluxed to prevent oxidation. Commercially prepared fluxes should be used. Though borax is widely used, it suffers the disadvantage that it effloresces (swells greatly) which can displace the pieces of solder and even the units. An antiflux such as graphite may be used to confine solder to the join.

5 The investment should be heated to a dull-red heat before introduction of the solder, which will otherwise oxidize and fail to flow over the casting. Ideally solder should liquefy at 50°C lower than the metals upon which it is to be used; this produces a strong joint without causing the components to melt.

6 Solder is introduced at the end of the join opposite to that to which the blow torch flame is directed, and capillary attraction draws it towards the flame.

7 The flame is removed immediately the solder flows. Most solders contain a small amount of zinc and tin which volatilize quickly when overheated, causing a deterioration in the physical properties.

8 Soldered castings should be bench cooled.

9 The grain structure of all soldered castings should be homogenized, and then hardened to produce the required properties (page 50).

LOCALIZING THE BRIDGE

Bridges may be localized in the mouth by the dental surgeon, or on a cast of the mouth in the laboratory.

Localizing in the mouth

1 After the units are prepared for soldering, they are tried in the mouth and checked for fit and occlusion, adjustments being made where necessary.

2 A wooden tongue spatula is used to mix impression plaster, which should completely encircle the spatula; it is then inserted into the mouth and placed over the occlusal surface of the assembled bridge. Every effort should be made to keep the layer of plaster as thin as possible and to prevent it penetrating the undercut areas of the adjacent teeth (Fig. 4.20).

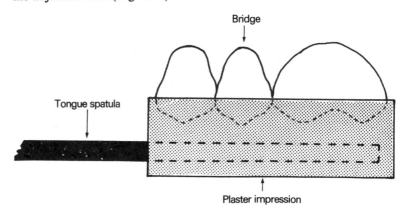

Fig. 4.20 Localizing a bridge using a wooden tongue spatula and impression plaster.

3 When set, the plaster and spatula are removed and the bridge units assembled before the bridge is sent to the laboratory.

Investing

1 Plater between the units is removed and the correctly seated units attached to the plaster using sticky wax. The joints to be soldered are filled with carding wax, to keep them free of investment.

2 Grease, oil or sodium alginate is used to lubricate the impression before boxing with carding wax. The box should be 5 mm wider than the bridge in all directions, but not larger.

3 Investment is puddled into the retainers using a wax knife, and then the box filled to its rim. Vibration of the investment is not recommended as this may dislodge the units.

4 When set, after about 20 minutes, first the plaster on the upper surface of the spatula is carefully removed and then the spatula itself. It is important to remove the plaster without damage to the investment. Removal of the plaster is begun at one end, a small cut being made from the centre of the bridge to the outer edge, then a further cut is made at right angles to the first. This small piece of plaster is gently prised off. The process is repeated until all the plaster has been removed to expose the occlusal surface of the casting. The investment is then prepared for soldering.

Localizing on the cast

1 The finished units are prepared for soldering, assembled on the localizing cast and sticky waxed together. A further piece of sticky wax, the length of the bridge, is softened and sealed along the occlusal surface. This forms a rigid unit strong enough to resist fracture during investing. The bridge is removed from the cast and wax run into the undersurface of the joint.

2 Investment is puddled into the retainers, the remainder being placed into a small wax box and the bridge inserted with the occlusal surface uppermost.

3 When the investment has set, the sticky wax is removed with a hot wax knife or rinsed with boiling water. The investment is then prepared for soldering.

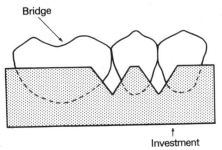

Fig. 4.21 Invested bridge. Investment is removed in the shape of a 'V' at the interstitial areas to allow access to the blowtorch flame.

Preparing the investment

The investment should be hand trimmed, with a wax knife, to a minimum thickness of 2 mm around the periphery of the bridge and 5 mm beneath it. At the same time investment should be removed in the shape of a 'V' at the interstitial areas, to allow the blow-torch flame to enter the join (Fig. 4.21). The investment is then heated, preferably in a furnace because it produces a uniform expansion with the minimum of distortion.

SOLDERING

1   The bridge is fluxed and then placed in a cold furnace, the temperature of which is raised to 700°C. Alternatively the bridge may be heated to 400°C in an oven, transferred to a furnace preheated to 700°C and heated for 15 minutes. A less accurate method is to heat the bridge over a Bunsen flame or with a blow torch.

2   The bridge is transferred to a preheated soldering block—a refractory block, the undersurface of which is saucer-shaped with a small rim to prevent heat loss during the soldering operation. A brush flame from a blow torch is immediately directed onto the assembly. When this reaches a dull-red heat, solder is introduced (see Appendix), the flame reduced to a pencil shape and directed onto the joint. If the temperature is correct the solder will flow immediately. Further solder is added until the joint has been filled, whereupon the flame is quickly removed to prevent overheating.

3   The assembly is bench cooled until the metal is a dull colour, when it is quenched to remove investment. The bridge is pickled, heat treated and polished.

Soldering bonded porcelain bridges

With high-fusing solder, bonded porcelain bridges may be soldered before application of the porcelain. With normal gold solders the soldering is carried out after porcelain application.

When using the *high-fusing solders* the bridge is localized and embedded in phosphate-bonded investment in the manner described previously. An oxygen–gas blow torch is set to a small flame with no hissing or sharp noise, and a solder melting in the region of 1150°C, which generally requires no fluxing, is used. The soldering operation is carried out as described for normal solders.

There are two ways of using the *low-fusing solders* once the porcelain has been bonded to the metal. Soldering may take place at the doorway of a porcelain furnace using a blow–torch flame, or it may take place inside the furnace. When using the *blow-torch method* the units are localized and sticky-waxed together, the porcelain facings are covered with modelling wax to prevent contact with the investment which roughens it, and the bridge invested leaving exposed only the joints to be joined. The work is then fluxed and heated in a furnace to 500°C, held at this temperature for 10 minutes to allow the wax to burn off, and then raised to 800°C. The blow-torch flame is set to a fine pencil shape. As the bridge is withdrawn to the doorway of the furnace the flame is directed onto the joint and the solder introduced. The solder will fuse immediately it touches the assembly. The bridge is left at the doorway of the furnace to cool. It should not be quenched because the porcelain would fracture.

The furnace technique requires the units to be waxed together but no wax is placed on the porcelain facings. During the investing procedure, no investment should be allowed to contact the facings. When investing has been completed short pieces of solder are prepared by melting one end to produce matchstick-shaped pieces about 5 mm long. The joints are fluxed (e.g. using Degussa 'T' flux), and the solder positioned with the ball end high up the joint and the other end resting on the investment (Fig. 4.22). It will remain in the upright position until it begins to flow. The work is slowly heated in the furnace to a temperature 50°C higher than the fusing range of the solder and is held at this temperature until the solder fuses. This takes about 3 minutes in an automatic furnace, but requires visual judgment in non-automatic furnaces. The work is allowed to cool in the doorway of the furnace.

The blow-torch technique is recommended when soldering a bonded-porcelain pontic to a gold bridge.

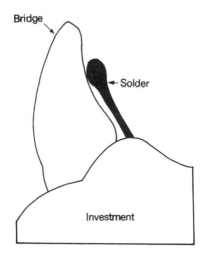

Fig. 4.22 Position and shape of solder when soldering a bonded porcelain bridge in the furnace.

Addition to contact area

Occasionally contact areas require building up in solder to correct faulty localization of the die or excessive polishing.

1   The restoration is prepared for soldering and the contact area isolated by surrounding it with an antiflux such as colloidal graphite. This prevents the solder damaging delicate margins or flowing onto the occlusal surface. When the antiflux is dry the margins are further protected from the heat of the blow torch by embedding in investment or wet asbestos. Bridges are always invested but, for small restorations, a 2·5 cm length of asbestos is moistened, folded into a roll and placed inside the restoration allowing the excess to overlap the margins. The asbestos is flattened to allow the restoration to lie on its side, keeping the contact area uppermost. Asbestos may be heated immediately, whereas investment takes 20 minutes to set and requires a slow heating process.

2   The work is fluxed and placed on a soldering block. The blow torch is held in the left hand and, with a brush flame, the work is heated to a dull-red heat. The flame is then reduced to a thin pencil shape and the solder placed on the work to complete the operation.

3   The restoration is quenched, pickled, polished and heat treated. The final contouring is carried out at the chairside.

Soldering a hole

When a hole has, by mistake, been ground through a casting it is difficult to solder because the area surrounding the hole, being thin,

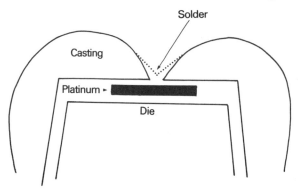

Fig. 4.23   Occlusal holes are difficult to solder. The best method is to adapt a piece of platinum foil to the die in the area of the hole and position the casting over it. The foil and casting are waxed together in readiness for investing and soldering.

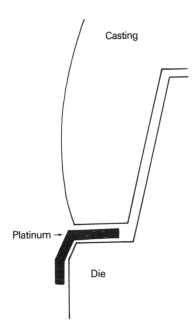

Casting

Platinum →

Die

Fig. 4.24 Repairing a deficient gingival margin. A piece of platinum foil is adapted to the margin of the die and waxed to the casting in readiness for investing and soldering.

melts when the blow-torch flame touches it, making the hole even bigger. Solder will not 'jump' such large gaps so it builds around the periphery of the hole instead of filling it. This is overcome as follows.

1 Antiflux is applied to the fitting surface of the prepared casting.

2 A piece of platinum foil is adapted to the die in the area of the hole and the casting seated over it (Fig. 4.23). The foil and casting are sticky-waxed together, wax being applied through the hole, and invested.

3 The restoration is heated and solder introduced. As it fuses it will flow over the surface of the foil to join it to the casting.

4 After quenching, the foil is removed from the fitting surface of the casting using a round bur. The thickness of the metal is checked with a pair of callipers and the restoration polished.

Repairing a deficient margin

A piece of platinum foil is adapted to the margin of the die and waxed to the casting (Fig. 4.24). This is invested and soldered in the manner described. After quenching, the foil is ground off and the margin recontoured and polished.

5 Porcelain Jacket Crown

Porcelain is a conglomerate of crystalline materials which when mixed together and fired are converted into an amorphous mass. The materials used in the formulation of porcelain are quartz, kaolin (or its equivalent), feldspar (or more recently nepheline syenite), alumina, fluxes such as lithia or potassium silicate and colouring agents in the form of metallic oxides (see Appendix). The manufacturer mixes and fires the constituents to bind them, and then finely grinds the mass into a frit. This frit is used to make the porcelain crown. Porcelain was introduced for the construction of jacket crowns in the latter half of the nineteenth century, but its low impact strength remained a problem for over half a century. With the introduction of vacuum-fired porcelain in the early fifties, it was hoped to overcome some of the deficiencies of the air-fired porcelains, but there were no improvements in the way of increased strength. In 1965 Hughes and McClean introduced aluminous porcelain which almost revolutionized jacket crown construction. This porcelain contains alumina (aluminium oxide, Al_2O_3) which prevents cracks developing within the porcelain. The base layer of porcelain, the core, contains 40% alumina (see Appendix). There are two types of aluminous porcelain available, air-fired and vacuum-fired, the principles of construction of each type being identical.

Matrix

The particles of porcelain are held together during the primary stages of jacket crown construction by water which evaporates during the firing cycle to leave the porcelain ready for fusing. To prevent the powder collapsing during the firing cycle it is built on a metal matrix which is a thin sheet of metal (0·02 mm thick) closely adapted to the die. It must be capable of withstanding the porcelain firing temperatures (1050°C) without distortion and remain chemically inert at these temperatures, for which reasons platinum is the material of choice.

The instruments required to form the matrix are a pair of college tweezers, a pair of straight scissors and a burnisher (Ash No. 2 or its equivalent).

1 Platinum foil is cut into diamond-shaped pieces using the template provided in each packet by the manufacturers. A piece is annealed in a Bunsen burner flame until it is cherry red in colour, and then allowed to cool.

2 The foil is held with the widest part of the diamond in the horizontal position between index finger and thumb of the left hand, the middle finger supporting the centre of the undersurface. The foil is brought under the proximal surface of the die with the labial surface facing the right, the shoulder of the die lying in the long axis (Fig. 5.1).

3 With the die and foil firmly pressed together, the left thumb is used to adapt the foil to the lingual surface of the die whilst the right

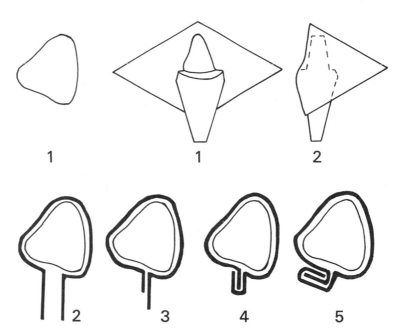

Fig. 5.1 The matrix. The stages involved when forming a tinman's or tinner's joint.

hand holds the dowel pin. Then the foil is adapted to the labial surface using the middle finger of the left hand. Pressure is maintained on the labial and lingual surfaces by the thumb and finger whilst the long points of the diamond are drawn to the centre of the proximal surface with a pair of college tweezers. The points are cut parallel to the proximal surface (Fig. 5.1) so that the labial extension of foil is double the length of the lingual extension (Fig. 5.1). The incisal edge is treated in the same manner. A triangle of foil is removed at the incisal corner where the proximal and incisal joins meet (Fig. 5.1).

4   At the proximal surface the longer extension of foil is bent over the shorter, first at right angles and then further to form a 'U' bend (Fig. 5.1). The two ends are pinched together using college tweezers. Then another bend is made to lay the join against the die, thereby covering the remaining free end of foil (Fig. 5.1). This is a tinner's (or tinman's) joint and it is repeated at the incisal edge.

5   The matrix must be closely adapted to the die. To prevent movement of the foil during adaptation it is held between finger and thumb on the incisal edge and apex of the die. The excess foil around the neck of the die is loosened and the foil is pressed onto the shoulder using the flat surface of a burnisher blade facing the die with its edge facing the shoulder. The extra metal required to cover the shoulder is drawn from the loosened excess. The foil is progressively adapted, trailing the point of the burnisher to prevent perforation of the foil. Although platinum quickly work-hardens it can be annealed repeatedly throughout the process. The foil is adapted further by laying the flat surface of the burnisher on the shoulder and moving it until the foil is closely fitting. Adaptation of the foil is completed by burnishing from the incisal edge to the shoulder.

6   The matrix is removed from the die. The excess metal below the shoulder (the apron) is trimmed to a length of 2 mm, following the contour of the shoulder. After a final annealing the adaptation of the foil is checked, special attention being given to the incisal edge. The apron must be a snug fit, excessive looseness being reduced by pinching the foil and flattening it against the die. The point of the tweezers should face the apex of the die to prevent cutting into the foil. The fit of the matrix entirely governs that of the finished crown and is very important because any deficiency of porcelain cannot be compensated for in the mouth.

SELECTING THE PORCELAIN

At least three powders are used to construct a crown: the core, the dentine shade and the enamel shade. The bottles containing the powders are numbered according to each manufacturer's formulae to produce their particular shades, and selected according to the manufacturer's recommendations.

Instruments

The instruments recommended to make a porcelain jacket crown are a clean Le Cron carver, a metal spatula, a large glass slab, a container for holding water and three sable brushes (Numbers 00, 3 and 10). A box of absorbent tissues, a clean razor blade and an assortment of diamond grinding instruments are also required.

Core

1   The teeth adjacent to the die on the master cast are coated with clear varnish or aeroplane dope.
2   The required core material is mixed, on a glass slab, with distilled water to form a thick paste. Distilled water, besides being free from foreign bodies, has a low viscosity and high surface tension which help when building a crown. An open container of distilled water for washing the brushes and a piece of sponge or absorbent tissue for drying them, are prepared.
3   A folded paper tissue is held ready between index and middle fingers of the left hand, to absorb moisture from the porcelain as it is built on the matrix, and the die between the index finger and thumb of the same hand (Fig. 5.2). A No. 3 sable brush is moistened, excess water being removed by wiping the brush on the sponge and, using the brush like a spatula, a small ball of porcelain is picked up and painted onto the labial surface of the matrix. It is important that the

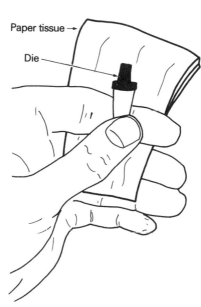

Paper tissue →

Die

Fig. 5.2   A folded tissue is held between index and middle fingers of the left hand and the die between index finger and thumb.

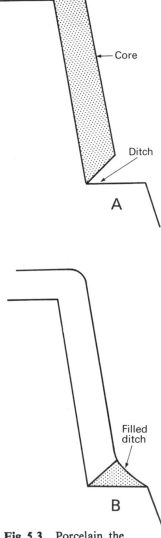

Fig. 5.3 Porcelain, the thickness of a fine pencil line is removed from the shoulder to form a ditch (A). This is later filled by flaring the core to the edge of the shoulder (B).

brush is washed between each application of porcelain. Further applications are made until the matrix has been completely covered. When the porcelain takes on a moist appearance, it is dried with the absorbent tissue held in the left hand. After building, the core is condensed by gently rubbing the serrations of a Le Cron carver across the apex of the die. As the excess moisture comes to the surface it should be absorbed.

4 The core is trimmed with a Le Cron carver to 0·5 mm which is half the width of the shoulder—a 20% firing contraction will reduce this to 0·4 mm. There is a tendency for contraction to distort the matrix at the shoulder. This is minimized by removing porcelain from the shoulder. Using the point of a Le Cron carver a line of porcelain, as thin as a pencil line, is removed from the shoulder to form a 'ditch', care being exercised to prevent penetration of the foil. A damp No. 00 brush is used to clean loose powder from the matrix. The ditch is filled after the first firing (Fig. 5.3).

5 The matrix is carefully removed from the die by holding the proximal surfaces of the crown between index finger and thumb of one hand, with the tips past the gingival margin, pointing towards the apex of the die. The die is held between finger and thumb of the other hand, their outline forming an oval shape. With the tips of both fingers of both hands in contact, the fingers holding the die are formed into a letter 'O' by which action the die is drawn out of the matrix (Fig. 5.4). The fitting surface of the matrix is brushed to remove every trace of loose powder and the crown placed on a crown stand in readiness for firing (see page 93).

6 After firing, the matrix is readapted to the die and the ditch filled, the core being flared to the edge of the shoulder (Fig. 5.3) and the porcelain condensed by vibration. Any fissures present are also filled. Porcelain on the apron is brushed off to finish the core exactly at the edge of the shoulder.

7 The crown is placed on a crown stand ready for firing.

Dentine and enamel

The shades of porcelain used for making the dentine and enamel portions of the porcelain crown are, for convenience, called simply 'dentine' and 'enamel'.

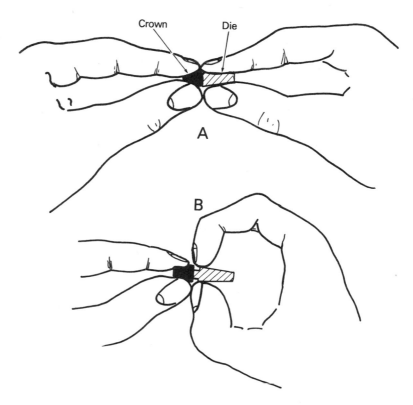

Fig. 5.4 Removing the die from the matrix. With the tips of the fingers of both hands in contact (A) the fingers holding the die are formed into the letter 'O' (B), by which action the die is withdrawn from the matrix.

1 The required powders are mixed to a thick paste. The crown is placed on the die in the master cast and the index finger of the left hand placed on the lingual surface of the core. A clean tissue is also held in the left hand. Using a brush in the manner described for the core, the whole of the labial surface is built in dentine; periodically the excess moisture is absorbed with a tissue. A moist brush is flicked along the proximal angles to prevent porcelain spreading onto the labial surface of the adjacent teeth. The labial contour is overbuilt by 0·5 mm, the incisal edge finishing at the height of the adjacent teeth.

2 The master cast is turned so that the lingual surface faces the operator and the lingual surface of the crown built in dentine.

3 When the labial and lingual surfaces have been built, the labial surface of the dentine shade of porcelain is chamfered from the incisal edge to the mid-third (Fig. 5.5) to accept the enamel shade

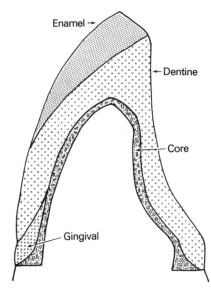

Enamel →

← Dentine

← Core

Gingival

Fig. 5.5 Porcelain jacket crown showing the position of the various layers of porcelain powder.

which is added by use of the technique already described. If the dentine shade is dry, it must be moistened before the enamel can be applied. The incisal edge is overbuilt by 1 mm.

4 Interproximal undercuts are cleared of porcelain and the die gently pressed out of the cast. Loose particles of porcelain are brushed off the crown with the large brush.

5 Finally the contact areas are overbuilt to compensate for contraction. They are lightly moistened, then 0·5 mm thicknesses of dentine and enamel are added to their appropriate areas and condensed by whipping with the large brush. Although overbuilt, the crown should resemble the desired finished contour.

6 The crown is placed on a crown stand in readiness for the firing sequence.

CONTOURING THE CROWN

The appearance of a crown depends upon a number of factors including its size, shape, colour, texture, mixtures of material, surface markings, fit at the gingival margin, relationship to other teeth and lip line. In this section, only the shape is considered and the following is a useful sequence to follow when obtaining this.

The proximal contacts are generally slightly oversize and this prevents the crown sitting on the die within the master cast. To overcome this the crown is placed on the die whilst out of the master cast. The proximal surfaces of the adjacent teeth on the cast are blackened with carbon from a pencil. When the die is returned to the cast the wide contacts of the crown will prevent it seating, (Fig. 5.6) the carbon on the adjacent teeth marking the high spots on the crown. These areas of the crown are removed with a diamond wheel, and the process of seating the crown repeated, the marked areas being removed each time until the crown accurately locates on the die within the master cast. The proximal contact of an anterior tooth generally lies within the incisal third in the natural dentition but it may be repositioned on a crown if this will give a better appearance, for example if placed more gingivally and towards the lingual surface a more squat appearance results, whereas placed

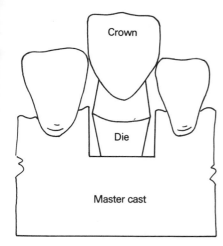

labially and towards the incisal edge the crown appears more slender.

The labial and lingual surfaces of the crown are trimmed to align them with the labial and lingual surfaces of the dental arch with a large diamond wheel. No labial characterization is incorporated at this stage.

The labial angles, formed where the labial surface meets the proximal surfaces, are crucial to the character of the tooth, their positions giving the illusion of a wide or a narrow tooth. If the labial angles run down the crown as straight lines the crown looks longer. If the angles are curved the crown looks less narrow. The angle is positioned by the formation of a chamfer from the labial surface to the contact area. The mesial chamfer is generally slight, the distal one is made more acute (Fig. 5.7). The chamfers are then rounded slightly to produce a natural appearance.

The cingulum. It should be remembered that the girth of the cingulum is smaller than the neck of the tooth which forms a slight outwards taper from the cingulum to the neck of the tooth.

The labial surface is now characterized. Labial developmental

Fig. 5.7 The effect of the labial angles on the appearance of a crown. Short angled are normal for most crowns (B), whilst as the length and acuteness of the angle increases a narrower appearance results (A and C).

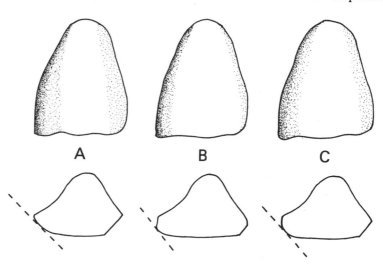

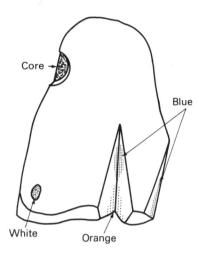

Core →

Blue

White

Orange

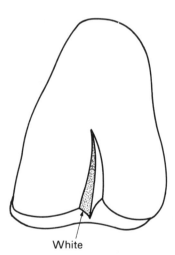

White

Fig. 5.8 Diagrammatic representation of the positioning of stains.

grooves are made and one or two small lines cut around the neck. Small cuts may be made at random over the surface of the crown, especially along the angles, to diffuse light and give the crown a natural appearance.

The crown is washed under running water to remove all traces of powder before it is returned to the furnace for glazing.

USE OF STAINS

The appearance of a crown can be improved by modification of the powders suggested by the manufacturer and by the addition of stains. Before modifications are attempted, it is a useful exercise to take some freshly extracted teeth and place them under water to study the colours present in the natural crown, and to note where the changes in colour occur. These colours become visible only when the crown is immersed in water.

Regular modifications are the use of a dark core zone at the neck, the recommended core material for the centre of the labial surface and a lighter one incisally. The dentine may also be altered in this way. Stains incorporated whilst the crown is being built can be effective (Fig. 5.8). The crown is built in dentine and enamel but not removed from the master cast until the stains have been added. The neck of the crown may be darkened by the addition of stain to body porcelain which is placed around the gingival area before the body porcelain is built (Fig. 5.5).

Enamel crack.   A razor blade is used to make an oblique cut in the labial surface and the porcelain is gently raised. The exposed surface is stained white and the displaced porcelain repositioned. The stain should be noticeable only to the operator.

Decalcification.   A small hollow is cut into the labial surface of the crown towards the incisal edge and the floor stained white. This is covered with either dentine or enamel depending upon the intensity of colour required.

Fillings are usually placed proximally in a half-moon shape. A depression is made and filled with core material which is covered with dentine or translucent porcelain, depending upon the intensity of colour required.

Incisal staining. A slight orange tint is often present towards the incisal edge in the developmental grooves of a natural crown. To simulate this a V-shaped section, tapering from the incisal edge to a point approximately halfway down the developmental groove, is removed. A trace of orange is painted towards the incisal edge and a little blue added along the groove to produce an illusion of translucency. It is covered with enamel or translucent porcelain. Blue is also added to the incisal corners to increase the effect of translucency. The incisal corners are removed, the stain placed on the lingual edge and covered with enamel or translucent porcelain.

Surface staining. A less effective method is staining of the surface of the finished crown. The stain is mixed with a special liquid supplied by the manufacturer and very lightly painted onto the crown, which is then glazed. This type of stain may be ground off if the effect is incorrect and repeated to obtain the desired effect. This is an effective method for progressively darkening the crown towards the neck, but not for adding the other stains described which should be placed under the surface for the best results.

FIRING SEQUENCES

Though many different furnaces are available there are only two basic types, those with vacuum pump and those without. Each manufacturer recommends firing cycles which should be followed for the best results, but a typical firing sequence for a vacuum furnace is as follows.

Core

1 The furnace is preheated to 1100°C and held at that temperature for 15 to 30 minutes.

2 The furnace door is opened and the temperature reduced to 850°C by either switching the furnace off or by adjusting the temperature control. Meanwhile, the core is dried in the doorway for 5 minutes.

3   The crown is placed on the firing tray inside the furnace for a further 2 minutes.

4   When the door is closed a minimum vacuum of 630 mm of mercury is obtained and the temperature raised to 1050°C. When this temperature is reached the vacuum is released and the crown removed. The time taken is 6–8 minutes, depending upon the age of the muffle (heating element), a new muffle taking a shorter time to rise.

5   The above procedure is repeated when firing the added portion in the ditch.

Dentine and enamel

1   The crown is dried in the open doorway of the furnace for 8 minutes whilst the temperature is allowed to drop to 750°C.

2   It is dried for a further 2 minutes inside the furnace.

3   A vacuum is produced and the temperature raised to 950°C, after which the vacuum is released and the crown removed.

Additions

The drying-out period varies from as little as 3 minutes for a small addition of porcelain to 8 minutes for a large addition. The drying-out period is followed by a further 2 minutes in the furnace before firing as described above. Very small additions should not be vacuumed, because the prefired porcelain may bubble at the surface, but large additions are vacuumed for the first 2 minutes and then firing is completed in air.

Glazing

The crown is preheated for 1 minute at the open doorway of the furnace and a further minute in the furnace before firing for $2\frac{1}{2}$ to 4 minutes at 960°C. The vacuum is not used when glazing.

Air firing

The firing sequences and temperatures are identical with those described above for a vacuum furnace, but with the omission of the vacuum.

REMOVAL OF THE MATRIX

In the past it was recommended that the foil should not be removed until the crown had been tried in the mouth. Nowadays the foil is removed before the crown is sent to the surgery. If the crown is modified at the chairside, it can be reglazed without distortion of the alumina core.

After the crown has been glazed it is soaked in water which seeps between the foil and porcelain. A pointed instrument is used to ease the foil away from the porcelain. Starting at the tinner's joint, the foil is pulled towards the centre of the crown. When it has been freed from the shoulder and walls it is held in a pair of college tweezers and twisted a little as it is pulled away from the incisal edge and out of the crown. The crown is then tried on the die, slight excess at the margins being removed with a hard rubber wheel.

ALUMINA INSERTS

According to McLean, pure alumina when incorporated in a crown increases the strength fivefold. This material is available as extruded curved strips, rods and tubes. Strips are used when the occlusion is close and in the construction of the all-porcelain bridge. Tubes are ideal for post crowns and pontics, whilst rods are used for bridges.

Alumina strip

Alumina strip is used on the lingual surface of the crown and is incorporated in the alumina core material.

1   A piece of the strip is shaped to fit the lingual side of the crown, about 1 mm narrower than the mesiodistal width and no higher than the incisal edge of the preparation (Fig. 5.9).
2   The core is built as described.
3   The alumina strip is moistened and seated into the lingual core material with a pair of college tweezers. Excess moisture is absorbed on a tissue. Discrepancies around the insert are filled with core material and the shoulder ditched.

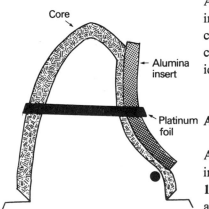

Fig. 5.9   An alumina sheet insert should not extend above the incisal edge of the preparation. It is held in position whilst firing by a strip of platinum foil.

4 Movement of the strip during the firing sequence is prevented by a piece of platinum foil 2 mm wide wrapped around the crown and finished with a tinner's joint (Fig. 5.9). This should be done with care to avoid damage to the core material. The core is fired in the normal way.

5 After removal of the platinum strip, the lingual surface is contoured, the matrix readapted to the shoulder and the ditch and fissures filled with core material. The crown is again fired.

6 The crown is then built in dentine and enamel, fired, and contoured as described. It is washed under running water, dried and a glazing medium painted onto the lingual insert. The crown is then glazed in the manner described.

Alumina tube post crown

The technique for construction of the post and spigot has been described in Chapter 2. The construction of the crown is described here.

1 The post is sticky waxed into the die, to prevent movement during the next stages, and the tube seated on the spigot and its fit checked.

2 The tube is removed and a platinum matrix adapted to the face of the die. A small cross is cut in the centre of a diamond of foil, which is placed over the spigot and adapted to the shoulder. Large 'tucks' are made in the apron to ensure that the foil is a snug fit to the die. The small diamonds of foil extending up the spigot are trimmed flush with the face of the die with a scalpel, and the apron trimmed as for a jacket crown (Fig. 5.10).

3 After the tube is repositioned over the spigot, it is sticky waxed to the foil and the top of the tube sealed with wax, care being taken that it is not waxed to the spigot. The tube, waxed to the foil, is removed from the die and filled with ceramic investment, a small diameter alumina rod being inserted into the tube to strengthen the investment. The investment should not extend onto the shoulder of the matrix. When set the investment is slowly dried at the open doorway of a porcelain furnace, and then heated to 950°C to burn off the wax.

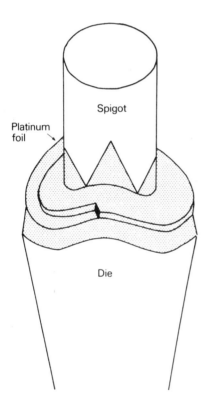

Fig. 5.10 Alumina tube post crown. After adapting the platinum foil to the shoulder, the triangular-shaped pieces extending up the spigot are removed.

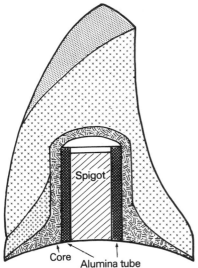

Fig. 5.11 A section through an alumina tube post crown.

4 After cooling, the top of the alumina tube is again sealed to prevent core material coming into contact with the investment, and core built approximately to the tooth shape. It is essential that the alumina tube is covered with core material (Fig. 5.11) to prevent its yellow colouring being visible through the crown. It is ditched and fired as described earlier.

5 When cool the foil is not readapted as before but the ditch is filled with core material and refired.

6 After cooling, the investment is placed in water and carefully removed from the crown which is thoroughly washed under running water. The crown is then placed on the die and contoured with diamond cutters. The foil is readapted to the shoulder, and fissures and the edge of the ditch are filled with core material. The shape is adjusted with core if necessary and the crown refired.

7 From this point the construction of the crown is as described for the jacket crown.

ALL-PORCELAIN BRIDGE

When aluminous porcelain was first introduced it was hoped that the material would prove strong enough for the construction of all-porcelain bridges, with no supporting metal. The appearance of such bridges is ideal but they eventually fracture because of stress set up by the independent movement of abutment teeth. However, when there is a single abutment this problem does not exist and in such a case the all-porcelain cantilever bridge has proved successful, provided that occlusal forces acting upon the bridge are small. Only this simple cantilever bridge will be described.

1 A matrix is adapted to the die, the core built and an alumina sheet inserted into the lingual surface. A small area of core material, the size of an alumina rod, is removed at the proximal incisal corner on the pontic side of the crown (Fig. 5.12) and the crown fired.

2 As earlier described, the ditch and any fissures present are filled. The crown is then fired again.

3 The crown and die are assembled in the master cast and a wax platform formed in the edentulous area for supporting an alumina rod which is cut shorter than the width of this area. The rod is seated

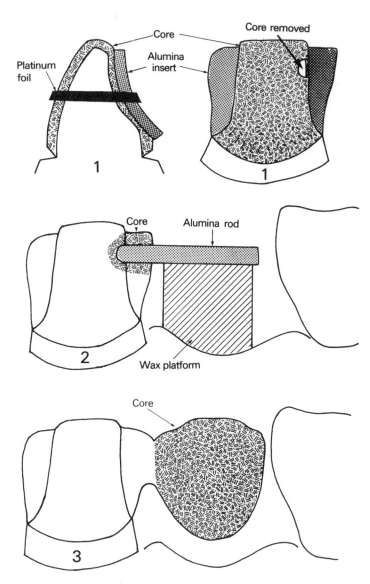

Fig. 5.12 The all-porcelain cantilever bridge. (1) An alumina sheet is incorporated on the lingual surface of the retainer and an area of core material removed at the incisolabial corner. (2) The alumina rod is supported on a wax platform whilst core material is used to attach it to the crown. (3) The alumina rod is covered with core material.

on the platform (Fig. 5.12) the lingual aspect waxed to the alumina sheet, and core material added to the labial surface of the rod.

4 The crown and rod are then removed and placed on a firing tray in a mound of silex crystals which support the rod. The core is refired.

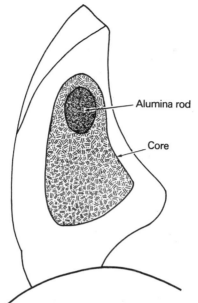

5 Core is added to the lingual surface of the rod and refired.

6 Core material is added to the rod in a tooth shape 1 mm smaller than the required finished shape in all dimensions, to facilitate the build of dentine and enamel (Fig. 5.12 and 5.13). This is again fired.

7 When the dentine and enamel have been shaped, the teeth are divided by running a razor blade down to the core interproximally. This limits contraction, preventing cracks forming across the crowns. After firing, the bridge is contoured and additions made where necessary, before refiring. The interproximal area requires careful contouring to prevent the bridge taking on the appearance of a single block of porcelain.

8 When ready for glazing, a line of black stain is painted along the proximal cleavage to produce the illusion of separate teeth (Fig. 5.14), after which the bridge is glazed.

Fig. 5.13 A section through the all-porcelain pontic showing the relationship of the alumina rod and core material to the finishing shape of the pontic.

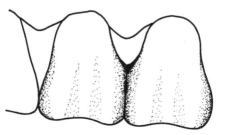

Fig. 5.14 The interproximal area requires careful contouring. A black stain produces an illusion of two individual teeth.

6 Porcelain Bonded to Metal

The technique of bonding porcelain to metal has been used since the early 1950s. The alloys first used were based on a high precious metal content, but chrome-nickel based alloys have been introduced in recent years. The bond is between oxides present in the porcelain and oxides which form on the metal surface during the firing stage. These restorations combine the strength of metal with the natural appearance of porcelain.

Tooth preparation

Ideally, the dental surgeon will have prepared the tooth by removing sufficient tooth substance to allow adequate space for both metal and porcelain. The ideal thickness of metal is 0·5 mm and of porcelain 1·0 mm. It is therefore necessary for 1·5 mm of labial tooth tissue to be removed (Fig. 6.1). However, this is not always possible and it is possible to construct a satisfactory restoration when only 1·0 mm space is available.

Impressions and casts

Compound or rubber-base impressions are taken and the appropriate casts poured as described in Chapter 1.

Types of substructure

The substructure is the metal to which the porcelain is bonded. It is shaped to withstand occlusal stresses and to permit the best possible appearance. The area onto which porcelain is fused is called the 'interface'.

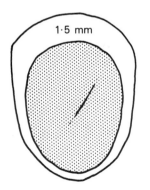

1·5 mm

Fig. 6.1 A labial shoulder 1·5 mm wide is required, decreasing proximally to a lingual chamfer.

100

Governing oral factor	Types of substructure	Comments
ANTERIOR TEETH		
Normal occlusion	Lingual gingival collar, full porcelain coverage (Fig. 6.2A)	Appearance excellent, lingual collar strengthens crown and forms lingual shoulder to which porcelain is finished
Heavy lingual occlusion	Lingual collar progressively increased over lingual surface until opposing teeth occlude on metal (Fig. 6.2B)	Appearance excellent until lingual collar rises above incisal edge of preparation, when translucency lost in preference to strength
Heavy incisal occlusion	Interface finished at incisal edge or in extreme cases 1 mm above porcelain level	Translucency lost at incisal edge
Proximal areas		
1 Single crown	Proximal area covered with porcelain (Fig. 6.2A)	Improves appearance
2 Bridge retainers	Interface normally finishes in contact area to allow for connector (Fig. 6.2C)	No metal should be visible when crown viewed from labial surface
3 Malpositioned teeth	Interface designed to finish at lingual angle	When tooth twisted in arch, exposed proximal surface should be covered with porcelain
POSTERIOR TEETH		
Normal occlusion	Full porcelain coverage with lingual collar (Fig. 6.2D)	Appearance good
Isolated heavy occlusal spots	Metal platforms incorporated on occlusal surface (Fig. 6.2E)	Metal and porcelain contoured to produce smooth occlusal table
Heavy occlusion	All-metal occlusal surface (Fig. 6.2F)	Normally used when minimal tooth tissue removed from occlusal surface
Minimal lingual tooth tissue removed	Lingual collar extended to occlusal surface	Often used in bridge work irrespective of amount of tooth tissue removed
Proximal area		
1 Normal occlusion	As for anterior crowns	
2 Bridge retainers	As for anterior bridge retainers	

Governing oral factor	Types of substructure	Comments
PONTICS		
Anterior pontics	Identical interfacial shape to bonded porcelain retainer but kept 1 mm away from tissue (Fig. 6.2C)	Allows porcelain-to-tissue contact and even shading throughout bridge
Posterior pontics	Identical interfacial shape to bonded porcelain retainer; metal occlusal platforms incorporated if necessary (Fig. 6.2G)	As for anterior pontics

Appearance is of primary importance near the front of the mouth. When space is available the entire substructure is covered with porcelain, leaving only a collar of metal at the lingual gingival margin to impart strength and produce a shoulder. Greater occlusal forces may make it advisable to increase the height of the collar along the lingual surface of the crown, and it may extend to the incisal edge or even onto the labial surface in some cases.

Where possible the interface should finish at the contact area to leave room for a connector (see Chapter 4).

At the back of the mouth appearance is most important in the buccal aspect of the upper teeth and the occlusal surfaces of the lower teeth. The buccal surfaces of the upper posterior teeth are shaped in the manner described for anterior teeth. The lingual surface is finished with a lingual collar which may extend to the occlusal surface.

When occlusal forces allow it, the occlusal surface is covered with porcelain. Though it is possible to have metal platforms placed within the porcelain of the occlusal surface, a heavy occlusion usually necessitates the whole of the occlusal surface being finished in metal. The proximal surface is constructed in the manner described for anterior teeth.

Pontic substructures are formed with the labial surface 1·5 mm smaller than the desired shape of the pontic when finished and the gingival surface approximately 1 mm away from the gingival tissue. This allows for porcelain coverage. The types of substructure are summarized in the table (see also Fig. 6.2).

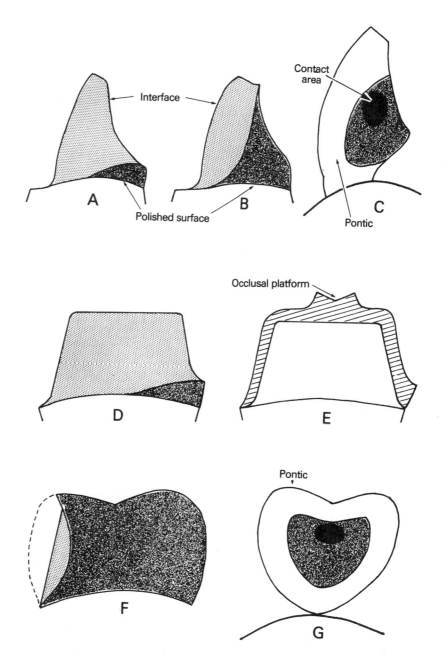

Fig. 6.2 Types of substructure (see table).

Pattern

The crown may be completely built in inlay wax to the required finished contour, and the labial surface carved back to form the interface. Because it is possible to see the shape of the finished crown before the interface is made, this is a useful method for the inexperienced operator. On the other hand, it is difficult to reduce the wax to an even thickness over the whole of the interface. This is a disadvantage because uneven thickness can produce distortion during the bonding of the porcelain, resulting in a crazed facing.

A more satisfactory method is the use of the thimble technique as described in Chapter 2 for veneer crowns, inlay wax being added to produce the required contours.

Selection of sheet casting wax

Ideally, wax used on the interface should be 0·55 mm thick which produces a 0·5 mm finished casting thickness. In practice, the wax thickness is adjusted according to the tooth reduction. Waxes of 0·4 mm thickness are average, whilst 0·25 mm is the minimum thickness acceptable if distortion is to be prevented. The wax should be 0·05 mm thicker than the required finished thickness of the casting to allow for thinning of the wax which occurs during adaptation, and for losses when the casting is being finished.

In extreme cases of incisal prominence, where a porcelain shading problem is envisaged, the wax is cut from this area but it should be borne in mind that a reduction in the interface area reduces the strength of the bond. At a later stage platinum foil is used to cover the hole whilst porcelain is built onto the interface; it is removed before cementation of the restoration.

Anterior crowns

1 An appropriate thickness of sheet casting wax is selected, normally 0·4 mm, the die lubricated and wax adapted to it, forming

a butt joint on the lingual surface which is sealed with wax. The incisal excess of wax on the lingual surface is removed whereas the excess on the labial side is folded over the incisal edge and sealed to the wax on the lingual surface (Fig. 6.3).

2 Wax is adapted to the shoulder with a curved burnisher, and the inner angle flushed with inlay wax, pressure being exerted to minimize contraction and to produce good definition of the fitting surface. The fitting surface is checked for accurate definition.

3 After lubrication of adjacent teeth, a further piece of casting wax is adapted to the lingual surface of the thimble. This is aligned to the adjacent teeth and then sealed to the thimble, the incisal edge being trimmed to the required height and the proximal edges trimmed.

4 The die is removed from the master cast and the proximal surfaces built and contoured with inlay wax. All sharp angles and grooves are eliminated from the interface to form a convex surface. The pattern is then sprued and invested.

5 Chrome-based castings fit more accurately when the wax pattern has been formed over a tin foil matrix. The matrix is finished short of the shoulder as for an acrylic jacket crown (Chapter 7) and is removed from the pattern before investing. These patterns should be annealed (see Chapter 2, page 33).

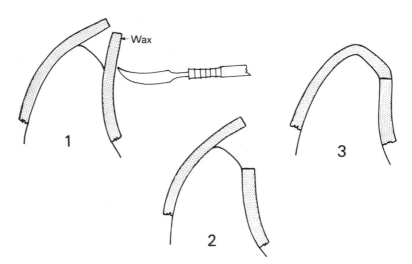

Fig. 6.3 Adapting sheet wax to the incisal edge of the die.

Posterior crowns

A full veneer thimble is formed, inlay wax being added to the lingual and occlusal surfaces as described in Chapter 2.

The junction between cusps and porcelain should be smooth and convex, especially when occlusal platforms are to be incorporated.

Pontics

1   Pontics are carved from a stick of inlay wax or wax is poured into silicone moulds (see page 60). In either instance the pattern is adjusted to the designs illustrated. Sufficient wax is removed from the labial surface to ensure a 1 mm minimum thickness of porcelain. When the retainers are bonded porcelain crowns, the interface of the pontic is made identical in shape to the substructure of the retainer producing an even thickness of porcelain throughout the bridge.

2   Localization of the pontic in the bridge is carried out in the manner described in Chapter 4.

The patterns are sprued, invested and cast as described in Chapters 2 and 3.

Primary finishing

Base metal alloy castings are sand blasted to remove surface investment and oxides. Precious metal-based alloys are generally finished as described for gold restorations (Chapter 3). Because the margins of precious-metal-based alloys are soft and are easily eroded, sand blasting, if undertaken, should be done carefully and sparingly. Polishing is with rubber wheels only, the final polish being postponed until after the bonding stage.

The interface is smoothed and shaped with pink alumina stones, and then rinsed under running water to remove dust. The interface of base-metal alloys is again sand blasted with a medium specially kept for this stage to avoid any trace of investment in the medium (see Appendix). Silica particles present in investment would fuse to the interface during the firing cycles, thereby reducing bond strength. Precious-metal alloys are normally rinsed under cold running water to remove debris and are then ready for the next stage.

Oxidizing the interface

Porcelain will not bond successfully unless an oxide layer is formed on the interface. This is accomplished by firing the substructure in a porcelain furnace preheated to 960°C. It is gradually inserted into the furnace over a period of 5 minutes. The lingual surface should face the muffle; an interfacial approach presenting the thinnest section of the casting might result in distortion. Precious-metal alloys are fired in air at 960°C for 10 minutes. Base-metal alloys are fired for 2 minutes under vacuum, then reblasted and fired twice more, making a total of three blastings and firings. After cooling the interface is closely examined for discoloration, light spots indicating traces of investment silica and dark spots indicating porosity, particularly in base-metal alloys. In either case the interface should be reground to remove stains, cleaned and reoxidized. When correctly oxidized the surface will be an even colour. The interface should not be handled after oxidation because the slightest deposit of grease or sweat prevents successful bonding. Tweezers or an inlay holder are used to hold the casting during the next stage.

Porcelain application

Only those porcelains specially designed for bonding onto metal should be used, the expansion properties of both materials being correctly matched (see Appendix).

Porcelains consist of opaque, dentine and enamel powders. Opaque powder contains oxides similar to those present on the interface which, when fired, bond chemically to the oxides on the metal. Opaque powder is built onto the interface to an even thickness of 0·2 to 0·4 mm and vibrated to obtain maximum condensation. Most manufacturers recommend the use of a single

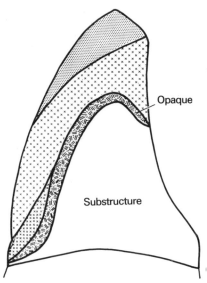

Fig. 6.4 A cross section through a bonded porcelain crown showing the position of the opaque layer of porcelain.

powder but this seldom produces the shade required. Better results are obtained by using the recommended shade of powder for the centre portion of the crown, a shade darker for the gingival area and a shade lighter for the incisal. Blue stain used sparingly at the incisal edge can produce an illusion of translucency, and pink in the centre of the labial surface makes the crown more 'life-like'. A great deal of experimentation is required to produce accurate shading.

Dentine and enamel powders are built in the manner described for porcelain jacket crowns (Fig. 6.4). Once the opaque layer has been fired the crown can be handled in the normal way.

Firing sequences

Most manufacturers recommend a drying-out period of between 5 and 15 minutes, depending upon the size of the restoration, bridges taking the maximum drying time.

A typical firing sequence for opaque is:

1 The furnace is preheated to 980°C and heat soaked for 30 minutes.

2 Whilst the porcelain is dried in the doorway of the furnace the temperature of the furnace is lowered to 850°C. A vacuum of 620 mm of mercury is then obtained and the temperature raised to 980°C to complete the firing cycle for precious-metal based alloys. Base-metal alloys are fired at 960°C for the first 2 minutes under vacuum and 5 minutes in air.

3 When fired the opaque should possess a slight sheen, bubbles indicating a dirty or porous interface. In such cases the opaque should be completely removed and the metal recleaned and oxidized.

A similar firing sequence for dentine and enamel is:

1 The furnace is preheated to and heat soaked at 960°C.

2 Whilst the porcelain is dried in the doorway of the furnace, which takes 8 minutes, the temperature of the furnace is lowered to 850°C.

3 A vacuum of 620 mm is then obtained and the temperature raised to 960°C at which temperature the vacuum is released and the crown removed from the furnace.

Bridges

When porcelain is applied to a bridge all the units are built at the same time, but separated into single teeth by being cut through the porcelain to the substructure at the connectors, thus preventing horizontal fissuring when the porcelain is fired. After the first firing further additions of porcelain are made to the proximal surfaces of each unit to improve its shape, before refiring. This improvement is repeated as often as necessary.

By staining of the embrasures each unit of the bridge is made to appear as a separate entity. Bridges should be carefully supported during all firing sequences to prevent warpage of the substructure.

Heat treatment

Precious-metal alloys are heat treated after the porcelain has been applied but before the final polish stage. They are heated in the furnace from 0°C to 550°C and kept at this temperature for 30 minutes before being removed from the furnace and allowed to cool slowly.

Final finish

Precious-metal alloys are polished as for gold alloys. Base-metal alloys are harder to finish, requiring all porcelain areas to be coated with sticky wax whilst the exposed metal is sand blasted to remove surface oxides. The wax is then removed by pouring boiling water over it, and the metal polished in the normal way.

7 Acrylic Jacket Crown

The use of acrylic resin for jacket crowns has been through a period of decline, partly because of the physical properties of the material and partly because of improvements in ceramics. However, with the introduction of newer materials its use for jacket crowns seems to be increasing again. Even so, many dental surgeons still believe that it should be used only as a temporary restorative material or as a facing on a metal substructure.

There are two ways of making the crown. The first is by forming it entirely in wax, and then flasking, packing and finishing in the same general way that acrylic dentures are made. The second is by incorporating a modified acrylic denture tooth on the labial surface of the wax before completion of the crown as in the first method.

In either case casts are made in the manner described for the construction of porcelain jacket crowns.

Wax pattern

1 Tin foil is used to construct a matrix, as already described for a porcelain jacket crown using platinum. Tin is a much easier material to handle. Also the matrix does not have an apron, being terminated at the inner angle of the shoulder.

2 Using a non-residual wax, the crown is built on the matrix which becomes an integral part of the pattern. The lingual surface is overbuilt by at least 1 mm (Fig. 7.1), which produces extra space in the mould to facilitate packing of the resin. After removal of the pattern from the master cast, a little wax is added to the contact areas to allow for loss of material during polishing, and to help compensate for shrinkage of the resin. The pattern is removed from the die and the position of the matrix checked to ensure that it has not moved.

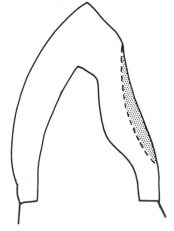

Fig. 7.1 Wax pattern for an acrylic jacket crown. The lingual surface is overbuilt by a minimum of 1 mm to facilitate packing the resin into the flask.

3 Both sections of a small crown flask are lubricated with petroleum jelly and a metal plate inserted into the deeper section, which is filled with dental stone. Some of this stone is vibrated into the crown which is placed in the flask, labial surface uppermost, at an angle of 20° to the base of the flask, and with the incisal edge level with the surface of the stone. The gingival margin is covered by a thick layer of stone to prevent it being damaged at the packing stage (Fig. 7.2). When set, the surface of the mould is lubricated with petroleum jelly, the flask assembled and plaster of Paris vibrated through the hole in the top of the flask.

4 When the plaster's exothermic reaction has warmed the flask, it is opened and the wax removed by pouring boiling water over it. Special attention should be paid to the gingival part of the lingual surface to ensure that all wax is removed.

5 When cold the mould is coated with sodium alginate, care being taken to avoid the tin foil, because sodium alginate here can cause a milky appearance in the finished crown, and avoiding excess at the gingival area.

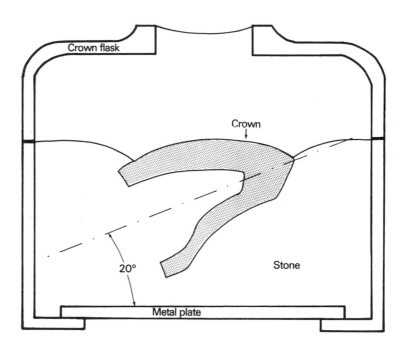

Fig. 7.2 The pattern is invested in a crown flask with the incisal edge level with the surface of the plaster and the crown at an angle of 20° to the base of the flask.

Packing

Acrylic resin can contract by up to 20% of its volume unless precautions are taken to reduce this. By using a polymer to monomer ratio of $3\frac{1}{2}$:1, allowing as much polymerization as possible to take place before packing, packing to excess and using spring pressure during the polymerization process, the contraction may be reduced to 5–7%.

Acrylic resin may be packed into the mould in the dry state or as a dough.

Dry method

1   Dentine polymer is vibrated into the lingual gingival part of the mould and moistened with monomer which is applied by a pipette. More polymer is vibrated in, followed by more monomer until the lingual surface has been filled completely. The labial surface is then built to excess in polymer only. The incisal edge is chamfered to accept the enamel polymer which is vibrated to blend the two shades of polymer, after which monomer is added. A thin sheet of clear polythene is placed over the resin, whilst it polymerizes to the dough stage, to prevent evaporation of the monomer which could result in a granular surface (evaporation porosity).

2   When the resin reaches the dough stage, the flask is assembled and its clamps applied to compress the resin. Before the flask is completely closed it is re-opened, any deficiency of resin made good, and then closed. The flask is opened once more and peripheral excess material (flash) removed.

3   Stains and characterizations are added in a similar manner to that already described for porcelain jacket crowns. Finally, the whole of the labial surface is covered with a sprinkling of clear polymer, which is moistened with monomer, covered with polythene and allowed to polymerize for a few minutes. The flask is then closed with the polythene still in position and the clamps securely tightened in readiness for the polymerization process. The disadvantage of this technique is the lack of control over the polymer–monomer ratio, and this might cause variations in the shade obtained between one crown and another.

Dough method

1 The correct shade of polymer is added to the monomer in the ratio $3\frac{1}{2}:1$, and allowed to polymerize to a soft dough in the pot, with the lid in place to prevent evaporation of monomer. The enamel is mixed 5 minutes after the dentine.

2 When the dentine reaches the stringy stage a small piece is rolled into a strip about 2·0 mm in diameter and is coaxed behind the stump with a burnisher or Le Cron carver, starting from one proximal surface and packing until the dough traverses the lingual surface and appears at the other proximal surface. This procedure prevents deficiency of acrylic at the shoulder of the crown on its lingual surface. More of the acrylic strip is added until the whole of the cavity on the lingual surface has been filled. This is easy to do when the lingual surface of the crown has been overbuilt at the wax stage. Having packed the lingual portion, the stump is also supported somewhat as it is compressed when the flask is later closed. Care should be taken throughout to prevent damage to the mould by packing instruments. Dentine is added to the labial surface, covered with polythene and the flask partly closed as described above.

3 The flask is opened, checked for adequate packing, the peripheral excess is removed and the incisal edge trimmed to accept the enamel resin. The enamel should be in a soft stringy state to prevent a demarcation line between the two resins, and the border is gently manipulated to blend the shades. The flask is closed and reopened when staining is added as required, the resin covered with clean polythene, and the flask clamped ready for polymerization.

Polymerization

The physical properties of acrylic jacket crowns are improved by polymerizing in the same manner as acrylic dentures.

1 The flask is placed in cold water, the temperature of which is raised to 60°C, where it is held for 30 minutes. The temperature is then raised to 70°C and held for 20 minutes, when the flask is removed and allowed to bench cool.

2 Alternatively, and preferably, the crown is polymerized by dry heat in a thermostatically controlled electric bath for between 12 and 18 hours. This method reduces the residual monomer and produces a hard surface to the crown.

Finishing

After polymerization the flask is bench cooled and then opened. A sharp tap on the plate in the base of the deeper half of the flask should remove the plaster block; an instrument is then used to cut plaster from the gingival margin. Saw cuts are made through the plaster to the crown and the plaster prised off the crown in the manner used to deflask a denture. The plaster and tin foil are carefully removed from inside the crown using a sharp-pointed instrument. Care should be taken when removing plaster at the shoulder; it should not be chipped away but the crown placed in a solution of sodium citrate for 12 hours to soften the plaster which can then be brushed off under running water. The excess acrylic resin (flash) is removed, using white acrylic grinding stones, and the lingual surface correctly contoured. Finally it is polished using a cloth polishing mop impregnated with Tripoli polishing compound. Pumice is not used on crowns, because its abrasiveness can damage the margins.

Stock denture tooth method

By using a stock denture tooth, the final shade of crown is guaranteed and can be approved in advance by the patient. To be really certain of the shade there is some advantage in having the tooth already hollowed out in the lingual surface. If an unground denture tooth is used, a shade darker than required is selected because its shade will be lightened when the tooth is hollowed.

1 Hollowing is achieved using a large fissure or round bur. The

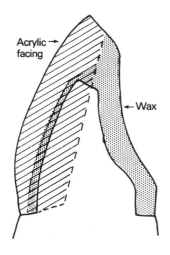

Fig. 7.3 The facing is fitted to the foiled die and the lingual aspect formed in wax.

finished facing should be approximately 1·5 mm thick with the proximal surfaces intact (Fig. 7.3).

2 After formation of the matrix, the facing is adjusted to fit the labial shoulder as closely as possible and aligned with the labial surfaces of the natural dentition.

3 The ground surface of the facing is coated with an opacifier, e.g. a solution of titanium oxide with the addition of colouring agents. This helps to reflect light to the observer's eye and the crown looks more vital.

4 The facing is then waxed to the matrix and the crown contoured in non-residual wax (Fig. 7.3). The lingual surface is waxed to its correct contour in this method.

5 The crown is invested in a crown flask with the lingual surface uppermost in this case. Extra care is taken to ensure that all the wax is removed from between the facing and the matrix. When cold, the mould is coated with sodium alginate and dentine packed into it. After a trial closure the flask is clamped and the crown polymerized.

6 The crown is finished as described earlier.

Bonding acrylic resin to a metal substructure

Acrylic resin may be bonded to a metal substructure of similar design as for bonded porcelain work (Chapter 6). The interface is coated with retention pearls as described in Chapter 4 (acrylic-faced pontics). The flasking, packing and finishing is as for acrylic jacket crowns.

Appendix

Page 5 **Electrodeposition of copper.** A typical electrolyte used in this technique is:

Copper sulphate	200 g
Sulphuric acid	30 ml
Absolute alcohol	2 ml
Distilled water	1 l

Reference:

PEYTON F.A. *et al.* (1971) *Restorative Dental Materials.* 4th edn. Mosby, St Louis

Page 5 **Cleaning the compound impression.** Surtenax (obtainable from Cannings) may be used to clean and degrease a compound impression.

Page 5 **Electroconductive media.** Silverpan may be used instead of Aquadag.

Page 10 **Die locating.** The device illustrated is the Flexico die locator.

Page 16 **Die hardeners.** Reference:

HOSODA H. (1962) Measurement and reinforcement of the superficial hardness of indirect stone models. *J. dent. Res.* **41,** Jul/Aug 752–759.

A typical mineral oil is Durusil. Care should be taken when using these solutions, as they can be a source of roughness on a finished casting. The pattern should be cleaned with a degreasing agent (Teepol) which is allowed to dry before the pattern is invested.

117

Page 26   **Retention pins.** Various types of plastic pin are available for use when constructing a pinlay, parallel-sided pins such as Precindent producing maximum retention. Reference:

KARLSTROM G. (1968) *The PRec-in-dent Technique.* Gävle, Sweden

Page 38   **Vacuum investing.** References:

MORRANT G.A. (1957) Vacuum investing and the use of a modified apparatus. *Dent. Pract.* **7,** 246–257.

ALLAN D.N. & MOORE J. (1962) Improved inlay investing vacuum bottle. *Brit. dent. J.,* **113,** 3, 85–87

Page 39   **Investments.** References:

ASGAR K. *et al.* (1955) Hygroscopic technique for inlay casting using controlled water additions. *J. pros. Dent.* **5,** 711–724

FUSAYAMA T. *et al.* (1961) Influences of clinical variables on a cristobalite investment. *J. pros. Dent.* **11,** 152–168

MAHLER D.B. & ADY A.B. (1960) Explanation of the hygroscopic setting expansion of dental gypsum products. *J. dent. Res.* **39,** 578–589

VAN AKEN, J. (1961) Distortion of wax patterns as influenced by setting and hygroscopic expansion of the investment (in English). *Tijdschrift voor Tandheelkunde* **68,** 8–9 (offprint)

Page 43   **Gold alloys.** Dental gold alloys are classified according to the American Dental Association Specification V.

Type I used for single surface inlays when the stresses are likely to be small and where burnishing may be desired.
Type II used when occlusal stresses are moderate, for all inlays and occasionally three-quarter crowns and pinlays.
Type III used when occlusal stresses are high, for three-quarter crowns, pinlays, shell crowns, all abutments in bridge work and pontics.
Type IV used when occlusal stresses are very high for abutments,

pontics and spring cantilever arms. Also used when casting intraradicular posts.

Page 41   **Fluxes.** Casting flux often consists of fused borax powder with boric acid powder. The author uses Deoxo casting flux.

Soldering flux consists of either borax glass, sodium pyroborate or sodium tetraborate with boric acid and silica. A borax–fluoride flux is used on nickel–chrome alloys.

Page 41   **Centrifugal casting machines.** The machine described in this book is the Krupps centrifugal casting machine (spring operated) Reference No. 41 201, with a cradle modified to accept small casting rings. There are many other machines most having different locking mechanisms, a typical one being a Nesor centrifugal casting machine Type A.

Page 45   **Electric arc apparatus.** The technique described is based on the Metromelt unit.

Page 50   **Polishing compounds.** The author prefers the Wipla-Weiss Universal-Polierpaste white polishing compound for polishing all restorations in the laboratory, followed by jeweller's rouge used in the block form.

Page 50   **Heat treatment of gold alloys.** For information on the theory of heat treatment of gold alloys refer to:

PHILLIPS R.W. (1973) *Skinner's Science of Dental Materials.* 7th edn. Saunders, Philadelphia and London

Page 56   **Temporary bridge.** Scutan may also be used as a temporary bridge material.

Page 60 and 106   **Silicone moulds.** These are useful for the production of wax patterns for pontics. A plaster cast of a suitable natural dentition or plastic teeth may be used as the pattern for the mould, which may consist of all anterior teeth or all posterior teeth. The base of the plaster cast is reduced until only 4 mm of the gingival plaster remains around the necks of the crowns. The cast is split to form posterior sections and anterior sections. Plastic teeth are set in 4 mm thick rods of modelling wax in two straight rows. Surface irregularities on the plaster patterns are corrected with modelling wax and the surface of the plaster sealed with sodium alginate.

Two rows of patterns are sealed, 4 mm apart to a small board or ceramic tile, and then boxed with modelling wax. The wax must be sealed to the board, be 5 mm away from the patterns and extend 10 mm above the occlusal surface of the patterns.

Silastomer* is placed in a suitable mixing vessel (the amount to be used will depend on the size of the patterns used). Sufficient catalyst is added to cover the surface of the Silastomer. These are thoroughly mixed and the syrupy mixture poured over the patterns to the top of the wax box. Setting time will depend upon the amount of catalyst added. After removal of the board, wax and pattern, the mould is ready for use.

Inlay wax is heated in a small ladle and poured into the mould until the necks of the teeth impressions in the mould have been covered. When set the wax is removed. It is useful to prepare a number of moulds giving a selection of sizes.

Page 63   **Porcelain glazing medium.** Two typical media are Steele's Super Glaze and the Biodent glazing medium.

Page 65   **'K' Pliers.** These are constructed from a pair of Ash solder tweezers No. 8 with a sliding lock. Two pieces of Germansilver plate 1 mm thick are prepared, one piece 5 mm × 10 mm, the other 10 mm × 10 mm. One arm of the tweezers is shortened by 10 mm and the smaller piece of German silver soldered a few degrees off the vertical position, narrow side across the tweezers, to its cut end. The longer piece of plate is soldered horizontally along the end of the other beak (Fig. A.1). The centre of this piece of metal is hollowed before the tweezers are polished.

Page 75   **Mandril for dovetail connector.** The blade of the mandril is first formed in inlay wax to the shape shown in the diagram (Fig. A.2). The measurements given are an average size. The pattern is sprued,

* Cold cure Silastomer No. 9161, Catalyst No. 9162; obtainable from: Hopkin & Williams Ltd. Chadwell Heath, Essex, England

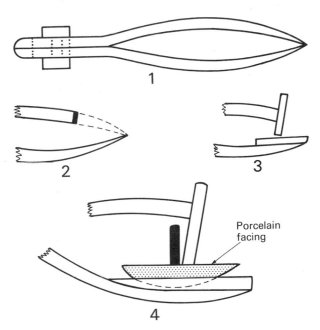

Fig. A.1   Stages in construction of 'K' pliers.

invested and cast in a silver–copper alloy, silver or chrome cobalt, after which it is cleaned and polished.

The wax mandril may be left long so that the finished casting can be placed in a lathe and a shaft formed out of the extension, or an independent shaft can be soldered to the mandril.

Page 80

Solders. Solders are classified according to their carat, fineness or melting temperature, and should have a melting temperature

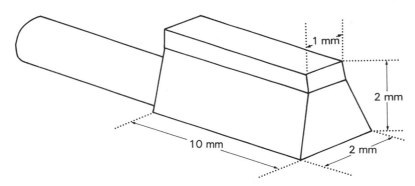

Fig. A.2   Metal matrix for a dovetail connector.

between 50–100°C lower than the melting temperature of the alloys on which they are to be used.

Page 84   **Colouring agents.** Reference:

JOHNSTON J.F., MUMFORD G. & DYKEMA R.W. (1967) *Modern Practice in Dental Ceramics.* Saunders, Philadelphia and London

Page 84   **Aluminous porcelain.** References:

McLEAN J.W. (1965) A higher strength porcelain for crown and bridgework. *Brit. dent. J.* **119,** 268–272

McLEAN J.W. & HUGHES T.H. (1965) The reinforcement of dental porcelain with ceramic oxides. *Brit. dent. J.* **119,** 251–267

McLEAN J.W. (1967) The alumina tube post crown. *Brit. dent. J.* **123,** 87–92

McLEAN J.W. (1967) High alumina ceramics for bridge pontic construction. *Brit. dent. J.* **123,** 571–577

Page 107   **Blasting media.** It is important that a silica-free blasting medium is used to clean the interface of chrome-based alloy substructures. Fine corundum such as Edelkorund (obtainable from Metrodent) is ideal.

Page 107   **Porcelain to metal bonding theory.** References:

SHELL J.S. & NIELSON J.P. (1962) Study of the Bond between Gold Alloy and Porcelain. *J. dent. Res.,* **41,** 6, Nov–Dec
Society

STANANOUGHT D. (1967) A study of the bonded porcelain technique. *Dent. Tech.* **3,** 22–28

General Reading List

COOMBE E.C. & SMITH D.C. (1964) Some properties of gypsum plasters. *Brit. dent. J.* **117,** 237–245

FUSAYAMA T. (1959) Factors and technique of precision casting. Parts 1 & 2. *J. pros. Dent.* **9,** 468–497

FUSAYAMA T. (1959) Technical procedures of precision casting. *J. pros. Dent.* **9,** 1037–1048

FUSAYAMA T. & IDE K. (1960) Casting shrinkage of certain dental alloys. *Bull. Tokyo med. dent. Univ.* **7,** 429–438

HOLLENBACK G.M. (1964) *Science and Technique of the Cast Restoration.* Kimpton, London

JOHNSTON J.F., PHILLIPS R.W. & DYKEMA R.M. (1965) *Modern Practice in Crown and Bridge Prosthodontics.* 2nd edn. Saunders, Philadelphia and London

NIELSON J.P. & TUCCILLO J.J. (1966) Grain size in cast gold alloys. *J. dent. res.* **45,** 3

TROXELL R.R. (1959) The polishing of gold castings. *J. pros. Dent.* **9,** 668–675

TUCCILLO J.J. & NIELSON J.P. (1964) Sprue design for cast gold alloys. *Dent. Lab. Review* Jun/Jul

TYLMAN S.D. (1970) *Theory and Practice of Crown and Fixed Partial Prosthodontics (Bridge).* 6th edn. Mosby, St Louis

WETTERSTROM E.T. (1966) An innovation in sprue design for ceramco castings. *Thermotrol Tech.* Sept/Oct Vol. 20, No. 4

Index

Index

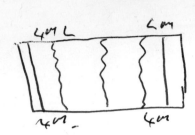